MW00632878

Praise for *Whole Body Vibration for Seniors*

Becky Chambers's new book explores everything you need to know about the many valuable health benefits that result from using a whole body vibration machine.

Written in an easy-to-read style, this book shows how using WBV supports the brain and elegant aging. If you are a curious senior, or you know a person who loves to learn about preventive ways to avoid health challenges, or you already have age-related disabilities, read this book.

—**Barry Taylor, ND,** author of *Love Your Body*
www.drbarrytaylor.com

I am so excited about this book, *Whole Body Vibration for Seniors*!

I am an acupuncturist, and number of years ago I was exploring whole body vibration machines, a process that soon became overwhelming. I was so fortunate to have come across Becky Chambers. She shared the knowledge and experience I needed to know to confidently share this extremely effective and powerful therapeutic and exercise system with my family and patients. I have seen firsthand the often-startling benefits that the proper use of WBV can bring.

WBV is powerful for both young and elderly. However, the benefits for the elderly to literally reverse common symptoms of aging can be astounding.

—**Jonathan Glass,** MAc, Ayurvedic practitioner, author of *Total Life Cleanse*
www.total lifecleanseonline.com

It is clear to me that this book will be the standard resource for why and how to use whole body vibration as a senior. From my work in a wellness center, I have seen WBV to be an excellent tool for everyone, but it is especially well-suited to people who aren't as active as they used to be. Ms. Chambers covers everything older people, or those who work with this population, need to know about WBV and in a beautifully organized, researched, and readable form.

As a therapist with a particular focus on neurophysiology, I know WBV to be a powerful tool for stimulating the brain.

Ms. Chambers is an authority in the WBV field. Her understanding comes from direct experience using this equipment for many years for her own healing, as well as with hundreds of clients of all ages.

> —**Robert E. Dallas, PhD**; founder of the Mind Spa, a center for neurological enhancement technologies; board member of *Conscious Life Journal*

Whole Body Vibration for Seniors is very needed in the marketplace, as we are getting positive results from our new Vibrant Health vibration machines, and great feedback from our clients, too! To share a few: "I've got more energy and strength to complete my housework and noticed the strength in my legs now going up my stairs in my home"; "WBV is helping me stay out of the chiropractors office for adjustments"; "I have lost eight pounds"; "I am feeling more balanced in my body"; "As a cancer survivor I am thrilled, as my bloodwork numbers improved for the first time in fifteen years. My doctor asked me what I was doing, and I told him WBV twice a week for only two months, he said, 'keep doing it.'"

As early boomers, our goal is to thrive in our senior years and to be more responsible for personal health. WBV is easy for us to accomplish, we can be in our street clothes and fit ten minutes in when we're out and about running errands. WBV is a positive solution for our well-being and positive aging!

Becky is so dedicated to her work and has helped so many people stay healthy and active! We appreciate her expertise and experience.

—**Joan Leavitt-West and Jane Leavitt-Arey,** creators/co-owners of Well-Being Studio, Twinsfeather, a well-being place, Bangor, Maine

I first came across the concept of WBV twenty-five years ago at a trade show when the first machines hit the market. At the time, I backed away from implementing it for two reasons: 1) initial platforms were prohibitively expensive; 2) no matter how hard I looked, I could find no good science to validate their benefits for osteoporosis. Periodically I would check again because I liked the concept. The results were always the same.

Then about three years ago, Becky Chambers's first book was lent to me by a patient. What a gift Becky has given us. Through her own experiences (personally and with clients), her diligence in interpreting the existing research and understanding of the differences in platforms, she has saved us much time, money, and effort. As a practitioner of now forty years, I recognized immediately the value of her contributions. Shortly after reading her first book, I contacted Becky and purchased a Vibrant Health Power 1000 for our Wellness Center and began to make them available to those who wished to purchase one. Our patients love it. A short while ago, a patient (now in her seventies) who had purchased her own reported back that her bone density had increased since using the platform (with no medication!).

Because a large percentage of my practice are now seniors (including me, LOL), I was excited to find that Becky has written a book specifically addressing WBV and seniors. What a perfect resource for our Wellness Center. Thank you, Becky.

—Patricia Salvitti, BS, DC

I love this book. Becky does a great job explaining how seniors can safely start and maintain a program using WBV. I have been working as a nurse in long-term care and post-acute care for twenty-five years and have witnessed firsthand the effects of the aging process, particularly related to sedentary lifestyles and poor health habits. So, I recognize the benefits of WBV for seniors. Use WBV now to prevent long-term care later.

—Marlaina Cataldi, RN, age 54

I'm excited about Becky's new book and have preordered several copies to give my patients. Once again, Becky has pulled important health information from the scientific community about the benefits of WBV therapy, condensed it, and put it into plain talk. I recommend WBV to my patients to elicit a measurable increase in strength, pain-free range of motion, and bone density. However, I cannot ignore the joy my patients express to me when they begin using WBV. I didn't expect such a response, but the happiness and energy of many previously sullen individuals is almost palpable to me after they begin vibration therapy. Better health and vitality over time isn't an accident, and WBV is one of the tools I provide to my patients for purposeful care of their future.

—**Donna Kost, DC,** Quad-State Chiropractic Clinic, LLC

In *Whole Body Vibration for Seniors*, Becky Chambers presents a compelling case that WBV could be an important part of healthcare for improving overall health for men and women. Plenty of research studies have shown WBV can lead to improvements in many areas: bone density, weight loss, muscle strength, mobility, energy levels, pain, and inflammation.

Becky's experience using this body, mind, and spirit therapy with people with health challenges, including herself, has allowed her to be uniquely successful in applying WBV to seniors. This book is an excellent buy for seniors considering whole body vibration, and a valuable contribution to the booming field of whole body vibration.

—**BoDanielle Park, MD, LAC, PHDOM**

Whole Body Vibration for Seniors is very needed in the marketplace. As an early boomer, my goal is to thrive in my senior years, and this is one of solutions to positive aging!

Becky is so dedicated to her work and has helped so many people to stay healthy and active!

—**Patricia Raskin,** media producer and host, Positive Aging programs

With Becky's help, I implemented whole body vibration in my chiropractic office as part of our patient rehabilitation.

WBV has helped many of my senior patients with a variety of conditions, including balance and coordination problems, plantar fasciitis, achilles tendonitis, low-back pain, bone health, circulation issues, concussion, and mild traumatic brain injury, among others.

I use WBV myself for brain activation, improved balance, feet treatment, low-back aches, and even with meditation!

I encourage you to try whole body vibration, but first, use her book as a guide!

—**Dr. Scott Fuller, DC,** author of *Happy Back,*
www.DrScottFuller.com
www.YouTube.com/DrScottFuller

After going through menopause, I was more irritable, woke up for two to three hours in the middle of the night, and had less of a libido. After using the WBV, my husband and I feel energized, stronger, and calmer—all at the same time. Our health has improved, and we both sleep peacefully through the night. We feel so much stronger that we can actually skip up two stairs at a time, and my husband is seventy years old. It has helped our sex life and libido.

We travel four to five days at least two times a month for work, and we notice a difference in how we feel when not able to use the WBV [machine]. We don't have the same energy, because when we get home and get on the WBV [machine], we feel an energized difference right away.

—**Geri Robak,** senior citizen

As a certified massage therapist, yoga instructor, and personal trainer, when I wanted a high-quality, affordable, vibration platform to use for myself and with my clients, I chose to buy one from Becky Chambers. When I wanted to become more knowledgeable on the power of vibration, I bought Becky's book (after reading strong reviews) and have since then shared the book with others and bought a second copy. As someone educated in health and fitness, I can vouch for Becky as a premier authority on whole body vibration.

—**Kentaro Ball, LMT, RYT CPT**

Whole Body Vibration for Seniors

Becky Chambers, BS, MEd

Transformations

Copyright © 2020 by Becky Chambers, BS, MEd

All rights reserved, including the right to reproduce this work in any form what-soever, without permission in writing from the author, except for brief passages in connection with a review.

This book is written as a source of information to educate the readers. It is not intended to replace medical advice or care, whether provided by a primary care physician, specialist, or other healthcare professional, including a licensed alternative medical practitioner. Please consult your doctor before beginning any form of health program. Neither the author nor the publisher shall be liable or responsible for any adverse effects arising from the use or application of any of the information contained herein, nor do they guarantee that everyone will benefit or be healed by these techniques or practices, nor are they responsible if individuals do not so benefit.

Cover design by Darryl Khalil
Interior design by Jane Hagaman
Models: Andrea Nichols, Diane Willmont, and Ula Zielińska
Model photos by Ryan Greeson, Maddie Freeman, and Becky Chambers
Author photo by Miranda Loud

Transformations
Lexington, MA

If you are unable to order this book from your local bookseller, you may order directly from the author at her website: www.BCVibrantHealth.com.

Library of Congress Control Number: 2019915746

ISBN 978-0-9890662-4-2
10 9 8 7 6 5 4 3 2 1

Printed on acid-free paper in the United States

To my mother and father,

who gave me my foundation and my wings

and who deserve a place in heaven

for their patience and faith in me.

"No problem can be solved

from the same level of

consciousness that created it."

—Albert Einstein

Contents

Why Vibe?

Only 10 percent of Americans get thirty minutes of exercise five days a week! Ninety percent are couch potatoes and have the same risk of heart attack as someone who smokes a pack a day. For overall health, exercise is at least as critical as sleep and good nutrition. Actually, the average American dies twenty years younger because of overall human misbehavior and willful ignoring of commonsense health habits.

Indeed, if you just stood and walked about three minutes six or seven times day, it would improve health and energy tremendously. More importantly, if you did vibratory movement exercise ten minutes daily, you would improve health, mood, weight, and energy and decrease risk of heart disease, diabetes, hypertension, obesity, osteoporosis, hip and knee replacement, arthritis, etc. Vibration improves circulation and digestion, reduces muscle and joint pain, and, most important, improves overall energy. It is even good for memory and decreases inflammation.

Watching TV does nothing to improve health or mood. In fact, if everyone threw out the TV and replaced it with a Vibe device (and used it), health and mood would improve more than any other change known. Although there are many other alternatives, such as Qi Gong, Tai Chi, etc., all of them take much more time and have fewer benefits than Vibe!

Walking briskly, biking, running, treadmill, racquetball, and many other exercises are all good, but the vibe device is at least as good and does more for all over health. One of my favorite cartoons says, "Which feels better, to exercise an hour a day or being dead 24 hours a day?" Are you ready for health and vitality?

C. Norman Shealy, MD, PhD,
creator of TENS, Gamma PEMF,
and author of *Conversations with G:
A Physician's Encounter with Heaven*

PREFACE

I have been using whole body vibration (WBV) for twenty years now, during which time I have become a senior citizen. I have seen WBV grow from a complete unknown in this country to a booming industry, and I am happy to have encouraged and been a part of that growth!

My journey with WBV began many years ago when I was unable to get well using Western medicine. At the same time, I have a strong scientific background, with a Bachelor of Science degree in biology, and six years of working in a research laboratory. After immersing myself in complementary medicine, I found a healing path that worked. Whole body vibration was central to my healing, and it turned me into an international expert and pioneer.

WBV seems deceptively simple, but it works on many levels— body, mind, and spirit—and to use it most effectively, you need to understand it on all of these levels.

I am a classic "canary in the mine." Forty-five years ago, my body began rebelling against the stresses of modern life by developing a host of chronic health issues. Those issues started when I was a young child with depression, which became chronic, at times severe, and continued for thirty years. I also had crippling insecurities and self-esteem issues. I developed addictive and emotional eating behaviors, including bulimia, and by my early twenties, I weighed two hundred pounds. By then, I also had rampant allergies, painful digestive problems, immune system weakness, and numerous disabling joint and nervous system disorders. Back then, I was an isolated freak of nature. Today, my experiences are becoming commonplace, as chronic health issues are skyrocketing. Forty-five years ago, I began my search for health and happiness.

Listen to my hard-earned knowledge and experience, and you may save yourself time, money, pain, and misery. You may even find joy, love, and success.

I began my search in my teens, using Western medicine and psychiatric care. For years, there was little progress, and by my early twenties, the physical complaints urgently demanded attention. I began to consider natural health, but by then so many systems in my body were involved and the situation was so complex that I was a difficult case.

For example, I had a severe case of *Candida* (yeast) overgrowth. This is a gut-flora disorder that, when severe, can become systemic, causing multiple symptoms and distress. I would improve with diet changes and products or drugs to control the yeast, but within weeks I would be sick again because I had become allergic to whatever product I was taking. Because of this extreme reactivity, I was called a "universal reactor" and eventually ended up allergic to more than three hundred different foods. For many years, I was only able to eat by taking daily allergy desensitization drops and rotating all foods so that no food was repeated within a five-day period.

I tried many different natural-health approaches and doctors: special diets, nutritional supplements, herbs, Chinese medicine, chiropractic care, acupuncture, homeopathy, heavy metal removal by intravenous and oral chelation, allergy desensitization, and more, but I was still going downhill. By my thirties, I could barely eat anything and had lost 80 pounds, ending up a slim 120 pounds of unhealthy, depressed, and lonely misery. My immune system was so overworked and weak that the slightest nick in my skin would inevitably lead to an infection that would take months to heal. My liver was so overwhelmed that I had developed multiple chemical sensitivity (MCS); I could eat only organic food and could not tolerate drugs of any sort. I figured I would eventually get some sort of serious infection, and because antibiotics only made me worse, I would probably die.

A key turning point came when I discovered whole body vibration (WBV) twenty years ago and experienced its potential to improve health. Using WBV in combination with nutrition, supplements, and homeopathy, I finally began to truly heal. Eventually, I began using WBV in my own natural healthcare consulting practice, Vibrant Health, becoming the first person in the northeast to use and supply WBV to the public. Without a doubt, WBV has enormous potential to help people, but like any powerful instrument, if it is used improperly, it can cause problems.

As a natural health practitioner, I have seen that WBV works best with an understanding of cutting-edge brain science, natural health concepts of nutrition, the impact of toxins on our bodies, and chi energy—our life force. I have written this book to help people, especially those older and otherwise challenged, to take advantage of the many benefits of WBV without stumbling into the pitfalls.

ACKNOWLEDGMENTS

There have been so many people over the last twenty years who have helped me to learn about whole body vibration and reach out to the world with this information. I'm sure I will miss some here, but my desire is to thank you all!

I want to thank all the medical professionals who helped me recover and learn about natural health methods, including whole body vibration (WBV). My experiences with my clients have also been invaluable, so a heartfelt thanks to all of you who, over the last twenty years, helped me to learn how to best use WBV to help others in need. Thank you, Dr. Jaswant Chaddha, for your help with my research, lending your medical and research expertise to the process, and for your belief and understanding.

Writing a book is a challenging process, so I appreciate and thank those who helped me put this book together, in particular, my content editor, Jeanne Mayell; copy editor, Tania Seymour; interior book designer, Jane Hagaman; and cover designer, Darryl Khalil. For the excellent photos of exercises and other positions on the vibration platform, thank you to photographers Ryan Greeson

and Maddie Freeman, and models Andrea Nichols, and Diane Willmont, and Ula Zielińska.

A heartfelt thanks also to my family and friends, who have provided support and encouragement throughout the years.

INTRODUCTION

Whole body vibration is well established for adults, particularly young adults and athletes, as an intense workout system and physical therapy system, but it may have its greatest impact in revolutionizing aging. All of the remarkable healing properties that have been shown to work for younger people can also work for the elderly, and then there is more. . . .

I have been successfully using whole body vibration with seniors for almost twenty years now. I routinely see rapid improvements in strength, energy, mobility, mood, and sleep, along with decreases in numerous types of pain. Whole body vibration is a true fountain of youth for seniors.

In a 2019 Vibrant Health survey of my customers over the past two years, 90 percent of whom were over the age of fifty and 64 percent over age sixty, they reported significant improvements in strength, energy, mobility, sleep, and mood (25, 28, 20, 17, and 14 percent, respectively). These improvements were rapid, often beginning immediately or within a few days of their first WBV session. At the same time, 74 percent of the survey respondents who

were in pain reported an average 52 percent decrease in pain levels—some while also decreasing their pain meds (a summary of all
the survey results is in the appendix). My vibration machines and method should be examined with double-blind research studies, but, until then, this survey can serve as an inspiration for seniors and as a guide to future research.

I have been successfully using whole body vibration with seniors for almost twenty years. I routinely see rapid improvements in strength, energy, mobility, mood, and sleep, along with decreases in pain. Whole body vibration is a true fountain of youth for seniors.

Of the published studies that have been done with seniors, some have shown encouraging results while others have not seen much change, but the researchers are not using the right approach. With the proper approach, seniors can achieve a youthful vigor and health they may not have felt in decades.

Researchers try to use whole body vibration (WBV) as a workout system for seniors, not realizing its powerful impact on the entire body. They end up using WBV with seniors like a bull in a china shop. As an older person, you need a different approach. Ours is a football culture where more is better, but the elderly are not a football players.

I have developed machines and a method designed especially for seniors. With this system, they can reverse health and aging issues that conventional knowledge and medicine say can't be helped—bone-density loss, decreasing energy, loss of libido, maybe even neurological diseases. Studies don't yet support WBV helping with MS and Parkinson's, but with a gentler machine and approach, perhaps WBV can help.

You are a senior now, and maybe you used to be very strong and had energy to spare, but perhaps there came a point when you hit a wall. You got a diagnosis, and the doctors said it can't be helped, you are just getting old. Well, in many cases, you can get better; you can use whole body vibration, and it can be success-ful—but not with the football culture–type machines. I will tell you how, and I will show you studies.

WBV has been shown by extensive research over forty years to be a form of intensive exercise. Movement is what we are designed for—it is the true fountain of youth, but it is often miss-ing from our busy and sedentary mod-ern lifestyles. As hard as it is to believe without actually experiencing it, ten minutes of WBV training will give you the benefits of one hour of conventional weightlifting, including increased muscle strength, bone density, flexibility, coordination, balance, and weight loss.

Ten minutes of WBV training will give you the benefits of one hour of conventional weightlifting, including increased muscle strength, bone density, flexibility, coordination, balance, and weight loss.

These benefits alone are enough to drive WBV's popularity, but, in fact, they are only the tip of the iceberg when it comes to the total effect on health and well-being.

WBV machines were initially invented in Russia for their space program in the 1970s to counteract the effects of zero gravity and as a training method for their Olympic athletes. In the 1990s, after the fall of the Iron Curtain, commercial machines were developed and rapidly spread throughout Europe. Ten years later, vibration machines arrived in California and began to be available across the United States. Currently WBV is predominately known and used for its dramatic effects on the musculoskeletal system, and there are many companies making vibration machines.

When you stand on a vibration plate, you can feel the vibrations going through your body with a sensation similar to a massage. It seems so simple, but every cell and molecule in your body vibrates, leading to a cascade of effects so astounding that I am regularly met with, "It's too good to be true!" It is true, though, and has been documented extensively by forty years of research. There are also millions of satisfied users worldwide, from youngsters to seniors, including: top athletes such as Shaquille O'Neal and Trace Armstrong; celebrities such as Madonna and Clint Eastwood; many health professionals, including chiropractors, physical therapy centers, and Dr. Norman Shealy (renowned pain specialist and holistic doctor); motivational experts such as Tony Robbins; and sports franchises such as the Denver Broncos and the Miami Dolphins.

When it comes to seniors and WBV, incorporating the wisdom of traditional healing methods with cutting-edge science leads to great success. In fact, when you know how to use WBV, it is particularly with older people and those with health challenges that you see the greatest improvements.

Western science and medicine approaches WBV with a narrow, mechanistic view of the body. This approach leads to poor results with seniors. Our bodies and minds work as a whole. Complementary medicine understands this, giving much more attention to the role of our thoughts and emotions. Nutrition and detoxification are also important, but they are so well accepted, with many resources already available to guide you, that I don't need to dwell on these subjects. I will cover these areas briefly, focusing more closely on mental stress and the power of our minds, which creates our energy, and how these elements interact with WBV.

When it comes to seniors and WBV, incorporating traditional healing methods with cutting-edge science leads to great success. In fact, it is particularly with older people and those with health challenges that you see the greatest improvements.

In recent years complementary medicine methods such as yoga, meditation, and acupuncture, which deal with our minds and energy, have been recognized as highly effective in numerous health areas, such as pain and inflammation, mental health, and immune system function. They have gained in popularity such that millions of Americans are enthusiastic users of these methods, and many Western medicine hospitals have complementary medicine clinics where these therapies are offered.

But an integrative medicine approach, where both Western science and complementary medicine are used, has not been taken with WBV research. Without this, the full promise of WBV will not be realized. On the positive side, this is a golden opportunity for a light to shine on the power of our minds—a unique force in our lives that deserves greater attention in medicine. Using an integrative approach, I have written this book to particularly help seniors, and others with health challenges, reap the benefits of WBV.

Chapter 1 focuses on the effects of vibration on your muscles. Involuntarily, all your muscle fibers will be activated, tightening and relaxing at the same speed the plate is vibrating—twenty to fifty times per second. That effect, plus the increase in gravity as your muscles hold your weight against the vibration, leads to a quick and surprisingly enjoyable workout.

In chapter 2, I look at one of the most hotly pursued goals of modern life, even for seniors: losing weight! We may have gained wisdom, but losing weight is now even harder. Don't despair, whether you want to lose a few pounds or a lot of weight, WBV can help. Like any exercise, WBV increases your metabolism and muscle strength, both of which help you burn more calories and lose weight. Just as important, WBV raises serotonin levels; this has powerful antidepressant effects and improves mood and sleep. Since many people overeat for emotional reasons rather than physical hunger, this effect can be a critical element in the battle to maintain and/or achieve a healthy weight.

Chapter 3 addresses the issue of bone-density loss and WBV's capacity to stimulate bone growth. WBV was, in fact, originally developed forty years ago in Russia to counteract the devastating effects of zero gravity on their cosmonauts in outer space. It turns out that vibration transmitted to the bones through muscle is a powerful signal to your body to increase bone density. For millions in this country and worldwide who are facing the dangers of weakened bones and the lack of safe and effective treatment, this is exciting news indeed.

Pain and inflammation are highly motivating! Luckily, used correctly, WBV is remarkably effective at rapidly and sometimes dramatically lowering pain, especially joint, muscle, and nerve pain. I have seen many people get on a vibration machine in pain and get off it a few minutes later with their pain reduced or even gone. Chapter 4 looks at this phenomenon and why the current scientific research is not able to reliably produce these kinds of results.

Chapter 5 is about the many life-changing ways WBV interacts with and affects the nervous system and brain. WBV rapidly raises the levels of two neurotransmitters, serotonin and norepinephrine, that have positive effects on mood and energy levels. In addition, exercise has been shown to be the most important factor for brain health, powerfully stimulating neural cell growth and strength. This is a godsend for everybody—certainly for people facing neurological disease and disability but for all of us really. Researchers have seen benefits from WBV for many neurological diseases, but there is room for improvement.

Chapter 5 will also look at the potential of WBV to help us by calming and synchronizing our stressed minds, helping us to move into a slower brain wave meditative state where our brain can focus on healing our bodies. Like acupuncture, WBV also works to stimulate your electromagnetic energy, now acknowledged by Western medicine as well as Eastern traditions as the basis of our neurological system and thus connected to all parts of our bodies. For example, like acupuncture, WBV often rapidly lowers pain and inflammation levels.

Chapter 6 focuses on common casualties of aging: energy, sex, beauty, and mobility. Feeling a lack of energy and zest? WBV may be just what you need. There are numerous physiological effects of WBV that increase energy, including raising levels of testosterone (linked to both men's and women's sexual libidos and energy levels). WBV also increases circulation, bringing nutrients and oxygen to all cells, and the antidepressant effect also sends new energy through your mind and body. The rejuvenating effects of WBV in all these areas can be attributed in part to increasing human growth hormone, the body's major repair, regrowth, and anti-aging hormone. This effect of WBV, plus the increases in testosterone, circulation, and electromagnetic energy, combine to give you a whole new lease on life.

In chapter 7, I address the role of toxins in health and how WBV helps your body to eliminate toxins. In fact, because WBV has such a powerful detoxification effect, it is usually the limiting factor for most people using WBV. I suggest caution; start slow, with just a minute or two, and increase slowly. In this case, truly, less is more—but can you imagine an exercise system where the biggest problem is not to do too much?!

In chapter 8, we will look at the plethora of WBV machines now available: what the parameters of the different machines are, what to look for, and what to avoid. Which machine is best for you?

Chapter 9 is a "how-to" section, giving you specific guidelines, gleaned from my twenty years of experience, for getting started with a WBV program. There is a day-by-day plan for beginners and tips for more challenging workouts for more advanced users. Included also is a guide to using WBV as physical therapy for numerous joint, muscle, or tendon injuries, and other types of disorders.

Read on to learn how you, too, can enjoy the remarkable rejuvenation and benefits of WBV!

CHAPTER 1

The Ten-Minute Workout

The Revolution of Whole Body Vibration

We are getting older . . . but this doesn't mean we can't still be strong and vital. Whole body vibration is here to help you!

One of the most important cornerstones of good health is exercise. As we get older, exercise is even more critical! We may tire more quickly, and we may not be able to exercise as easily, but exercise remains an essential part of good health. As seniors, more than ever we need the rejuvenation and regeneration that exercise stimulates.

Exercise: The Fountain of Youth

Our bodies are designed for physical activity, and they thrive on it. For example, exercise increases your circulation, bringing essential nutrients and oxygen to every part of your body, including your brain, and removing waste products. Ramping up this process helps every cell and organ in your body to function at a higher level. Just by exercising, you increase your body's ability to drive the circulatory system. Your heart, which pumps your blood through the arteries on its outgoing journey, becomes stronger. Exercising builds more muscle, which in turn massages the veins in the gentler but essential pumping action that moves the blood on its return trip to the heart. Exercise, whether in a more traditional form or now with whole body vibration, is also critical to maintaining muscle tone, bone density, and a healthy weight.

Exercise and Your Brain

Just as important, exercise helps your mood and brain. If you are so depressed and lethargic that you can barely get out of your chair and exercise, sometimes your whole life can seem like an insurmountable mountain. The good news is that the very act of exercising will increase the levels of natural feel-good chemicals in your brain called neurotransmitters; this will raise your spirits, energize you, and help your brain to function better. Plus, exercise has been shown to increase the number of neurons and neural connections in your brain. These are important components of intelligence, so you will actually be getting smarter as you exercise. Chapter 5 will go into much more detail about how whole body vibration (WBV) affects the brain.

WBV is a very effective and quick exercise. In hundreds of research studies, it has been shown to result in rapid increases in strength.

The Ten-Minute Workout

Whole body vibration (WBV) is a very effective and quick exercise. In hundreds of research studies, WBV has been shown to result in rapid increases in strength.[1] In fact, WBV was originally developed because of its intense workout effect over forty years ago in Russia for their Olympic athletes and space program, and it is currently used widely by athletes around the world, from amateur athletes to top athletes and sports franchises and teams. Originally studied primarily with athletes and healthy young people, more recent studies have also shown promising results with older people.[2-6]

Ten minutes of WBV provides an intense, full-body workout with the benefits of conventional weightlifting.

Ten minutes of WBV provides an intense, full-body workout with the benefits of conventional weightlifting.

At first this may seem impossible, just too good to be true; but it is true—for young athletes. Ten minutes of WBV, however, is not an advisable way for seniors to start a WBV program. Seniors can gain great benefits, including strength, from WBV, but it is wise for seniors to start more slowly, with a gentler machine, less time, and a low speed, gradually increasing both (see chapter 9 for a detailed day-by-day plan). The exact workout effect depends on which machine you use and how you use it, and your workout should be tailored for your body and health. Nevertheless, forty years of research and the devotion of thousands of professional athletes and elite users, attest to WBV's effectiveness.

How Whole Body Vibration Creates Intensive Exercise

♦ Holding weight against vibration increases the effects of gravity. Because of this physical reality (described mathematically as gravity equals mass times acceleration), when vibrating, your muscles must hold up to three times your actual weight, the exact amount depending on the amplitude and frequency of the vibration. If you have any doubt about this, consider the arm and shoulder muscle development of men who operate jackhammers.

♦ Every muscle fiber will automatically tense and relax at the same rate that the machine is vibrating, usually twenty to fifty times per second. That adds up to one thousand to three thousand little tiny "reps" per minute—much more work for your muscles than holding a static position (isometric exercise) or typical repetition workouts.

♦ One hundred percent of your muscles will be working, while in traditional exercises, only some of your muscles are engaged. For example, in a nonvibrating squat, only about 40 percent of your leg muscles are working, but if you are vibrating, 100 percent of your leg muscles will be firing.

The combination of these three factors results in an intensive workout, in which, by the end of one minute, your muscles may be begging for relief. If the WBV workout is still not hard enough for you, you can also carry weights, which will rapidly increase the effort as the gravitational increase from the vibration will double or triple any weight increase.

You can also vary the type of exercise position to change which muscle groups must work to hold your weight. For example, you can do push-ups for upper-body strength, or sit on the plate in a V shape (see page 167) to work the abdominal muscles. There are endless variations in position to engage different muscle groups. A typical workout includes one-minute intervals in numerous different positions to achieve the effect of a full-body workout in ten minutes.

While circulation does increase with WBV, this is partly due to the massaging action of the muscle fibers as they tense and relax. WBV does not provide intensive aerobic exercise, so you should also incorporate some type of aerobic exercise into your total fitness plan, such as walking, biking, running, swimming, etc. You will probably find it much easier to do this when you are using WBV because of the powerful energizing and mood-elevating effects of vibration.

And while WBV is an intensive workout for your muscles, most people will not break into a sweat—so you don't even need to change your clothes

Holding weight against vibration increases the effects of gravity. Every muscle fiber will automatically tense and relax at the same rate that the machine is vibrating. One hundred percent of your muscle will be working, while in traditional exercises, only some of your muscles are engaged.

or take a shower! Just hop onto your vibration plate for five to ten minutes, whenever is convenient. Everybody can fit five to ten minutes a day into their life.

TESTIMONIALS

After many years of intense stress, I was so overwhelmed and exhausted that I had to break up my tasks into manageable pieces. Going out of the house was accomplished with great effort. Then I started using Becky's vibrating platforms. These platforms were the key to my building up my strength to do daily tasks. All I did was stand for five minutes, holding on to the curved bar on the gentle one; then later I moved to the Power 1000 platform, sometimes holding the straps for balance and now for strength training. Once, all I could do was my five minutes of vibration in a day; now I find myself working in my garden for short periods of time, going to the grocery, and now able to do more than one thing in the same day. Not exaggerating, I have my "no problem, I can do it" attitude back, with an "edit myself" approach of not trying to do quite as much as I once did. The vibration platform makes the rest of my health routine work.

—Mary, age 69, registered nurse

My back muscles and posture have been uneven for thirty years due to scoliosis. Whole body vibration has helped to even out my upper-body muscle strength and mass, especially on my left side where it was weaker. I am standing straighter now. It also helps my sinuses drain and my lungs feel less congested. I use it especially in the winter to stay more physically active, and it has a nice massage-like affect. I am still working and very active, and I'm determined to stay that way.

—*Bill, age 72*

I was mountain biking in the fall of 2017, hit a root, fell off my bike, hit the ground, and fractured my little finger. In the fall of 2018, after using my WBV machine for about four months, I was mountain biking in the same woods and hit a root. This time, as my bike was falling, I was able to jump off and land on my feet. I felt very strong and in control, increased core strength and balance, quad and calf strength. I felt great! I felt like I was an agile twenty-year-old again. Also, a year after using the Vibrant Health Power 1000 vibration machine, my calves were bigger, evidenced by my ski boot buckles needing to be adjusted!

This past ski season in 2019, I had a serious ski fall that could've been deadly; however, no major injuries, no broken bones, and my body healed quickly from bruises and sore muscles and knee! I was fifty-three at the time but felt like a young athlete.

Additionally, I want to mention that going through menopause is a great time to use the WBV machine as it helps to maintain muscle tone, which in turn helps boost mood and body image as things begin to shift from changes in hormones.

—*Marliana Cataldi, RN, age 54*

Recent research has been less exciting, however, as researchers have tried to pin down exactly how to best use WBV with older people, especially those with health issues. There is no doubt that

WBV is intensive exercise, but research is conflicted, in situations such as arthritis, on whether it is better than conventional exercise.[7, 8]

I believe the problem with research on seniors is that it is not being done properly. Using the knowledge gained from a lifetime of dealing with health issues, with many corollaries to those of seniors, I have great success using WBV for seniors with health issues. In fact, older, ill, and otherwise less fit and strong people are the very people most likely to see dramatic improvements.

TESTIMONIAL

I am sixty-eight years young and have had several chronic diagnoses for over thirty years. After over a year of immobility due to low back stenosis pain and chronic hip issues, my biggest concerns were loss of ability, endurance, and vitality. Conventional treatments were not geared for my age and disability from chronic conditions. In the spring of 2018, I started using Becky's Gentle 500 vibration machine. I felt a boost of confidence in my body and myself as I gained energy and my pain decreased. I consulted with Becky again and upgraded to the Vibrant Health Power 1000 in January 2019. I used to think I was going to end up in a wheelchair; now I am swimming every other day, and I recently added using a light weight-lifting machine routine to my gym workouts. The increased confidence from my growing endurance and strength is priceless.

I am forever grateful to have found my way to whole body vibration and Becky.

—Sandy Gong, age 68

WBV Research with Seniors

While the intense muscle strengthening effect of WBV is clear, recent scientific research with older people with health problems has resulted in confusing and contradictory results. For example, in a 2016 systematic review[i] of four research studies on quadriceps (thigh muscle) strength in older women with knee osteoarthritis, the authors concluded that "only one found significantly greater quadriceps muscle strength gains" from using WBV than from regular exercise.[9]

But, while researchers have adapted WBV programs to seniors to some degree, I do not believe they have gone far enough. Most of the WBV research done with seniors has been done with the same types of machines that have been used with young people and athletes. Less strenuous workout protocols are used, but they are still considerably more intense than my experience and research has shown is best. For older people with stressed bodies and often dealing with health challenges, the best approach is a gentle approach.

Powerful machines delivering high amplitude and high gravitational force (g-force) vibration, often at high frequencies, were used in all four of the studies in that 2016 review of strength and knee osteoarthritis. (See chapter 8 for a full explanation of the different types of machines and parameters of vibration.) Combined with greater time spent working out on the vibration plate than I recommend, this kind of a program results in a high intensity workout that is too much for seniors with health issues.

---

[i]Considered the gold standard of research and typically, therefore, given the most attention.

Three of those research studies gave participants ten to thirty minutes of vibration on machines delivering vibration of 2–5 mm amplitude. The fourth study, the one that did report an increase in strength, started with three minutes of WBV and worked up to ten minutes over eight weeks. This fourth study did not specify the amplitude, but I suspect that it was high (as most studies are using high amplitude vibration) and that the results would likely have been better if it had been low. Three studies did not report g-force (a measure of the intensity of the experience, as it combines frequency and amplitude). The lack of amplitude and g-force data is an indication of the lack of understanding regarding the importance of this factor.

In contrast, I recommend that older people (and anyone with health challenges) start with thirty to sixty *seconds*, with vibration at a maximum of 3 mm amplitude, and then slowly build up the time and intensity of their WBV session.[ii] These differences may not sound large to people who have not been on these machines, but it is the difference between feeling like you are hanging on to a jackhammer and feeling like you are a powerful, purring cheetah.

There are also more factors involved in success with WBV than just a workout for the muscles. Particularly, WBV has a huge effect on the brain (see also chapter 5). It is in large part because of these other factors that it is so critical to go slowly and gently with WBV. Using my methods, I regularly see huge increases in strength for seniors.

[ii]My recommendations are conservative—they are designed to help everybody succeed. One can always increase the amount of vibration, but too much vibration can make you feel worse instead of better; so a conservative approach is wise, especially in the beginning.

Vibrant Health's WBV Survey Strength Results

In 2019, Vibrant Health conducted a research survey[10] of our customers using Vibrant Health's Power 1000 machine, which comes with a user manual containing the author's recommendations on how to use the machine. (These recommendations are included in this book in chapter 9.) Ninety percent of the respondents to Vibrant Health's survey were over fifty years of age, 62 percent were sixty to eighty years old. The survey included fifty-three respondents.

We asked VH Power 1000 users to rate their strength before and after beginning their WBV program on a scale of 1–5, where 1 equals "Very Weak" and 5 equals "Very Strong." On average, respondents reported a 25 percent increase in their strength and a 28 percent increase in energy within weeks of beginning their WBV program. Almost 20 percent of respondents reported increased strength within a few days of beginning WBV, 49 percent within one month.

Respondents reported a 25 percent increase in their strength and a 28 percent increase in energy within weeks of beginning their WBV program. Almost 20 percent reported increased strength within a few days, 49 percent within one month.

Testimonials

When I first started vibration therapy, I was so chronically fatigued that I would get a cart at the supermarket to lean on while I walked around, even if I only needed one item. After every vibration session (two per week), I felt stronger and energized; I was noticeably gaining vigor by the week. Two months into the therapy, there was a snowstorm that dropped a half a foot of snow overnight. I was late to my vibration appointment that day, because first I had to shovel out my driveway, and then I shoveled out my neighbor's driveway, as she is frail and elderly.

—*Ellen, age 57*

I had been vibrating just a few times when I went home after my three or four minutes of vibration, and I had so much energy I started scrubbing the kitchen floor by hand. When I finished with the floor, I started in on the walls. My husband, who was half asleep on the couch where we would usually both be after a long day at work, said to me, "What has gotten into you?"

—*Marianne L., age 54*

I have struggled for years with chronic fatigue. The morning after my first one-minute session, I jumped out of bed for the first time in about twenty years, plus my mind is clear and focused.

—*Jessica W., age 63*

How could so little exercise result in such a dramatic increase in strength? Because vibration is not just about making your muscles work. WBV researchers have approached the issue this way, but

WBV is also affecting every part of your body—cells, organs, nervous system, and brain—all of which affects your strength.

Getting Started with Your Workout

WBV is a quick, highly adaptable workout that can be tailored to any level of fitness: from the couch potato to the occasional jogger, the tennis player to the weekend warrior, or the amateur athlete.

For seniors with any type of health issue, it is best to start with just a very small amount of vibration (thirty seconds to one minute), and there is no need to do anything more than just stand on the gently vibrating plate. This will feel something like a massage, but through the involuntary automatic activation of your nervous system, and thus your muscles, you will still be experiencing a mild workout, and your entire body and nervous system will be stimulated to wake up.

Gradually and slowly, listening to your body as you go, you can increase the intensity of your vibration workouts by increasing the time and frequency settings. You can also add in different exercise positions that will intensify the workout effect. The end result: You will quickly start feeling stronger and better, and soon you will be doing a ten-minute workout that gives you the benefits of an hour of conventional exercise.

Note: See chapter 9 for more details, a daily plan, and photos of different exercises, massage positions, and stretching positions. For videos with exercise types and an exercise poster, see www.BCVibrantHealth.com and Becky's YouTube channel (VibrantHealthBecky).

CHAPTER 2

Losing Weight with Whole Body Vibration

Losing weight is hard . . . but losing weight when you are older is even harder! Hormones have shifted, we're not as active, our metabolisms have slowed down, and exercising is more difficult. The result is stubborn weight gain that resists our best efforts. Luckily, we are also smart! We have our many years of experience and wisdom to guide us, and now you have a powerful new tool to help you also—whole body vibration.

Why Vibration?

Whole body vibration (WBV) can help you lose weight and keep it off long-term by speeding up your metabolism, increasing energy levels, elevating your mood, and strengthening muscles—all in a short ten to fifteen minutes of exercising on a vibration plate. My own research and experience show that even if all you do is stand on the plate, you are still getting many benefits, including help in losing weight. Now you might be laughing and making a joke about those vibrating belts from the 1960s, but don't let the laughter stop you!

A 2018 systematic review[1] of eighteen research articles, with a combined total of 321 human subjects, looked at using WBV with obese patients. The results showed increased metabolism and weight and fat loss, along with improvements in other issues known to be related to obesity, such as heart health, peripheral and central circulation, glucose regulation, and inflammation levels. My own research and extensive experience with clients and myself also make it clear that WBV is a huge plus in any weight-loss program.

In Vibrant Health's 2019 survey of our customers, 50 percent of those who wanted to lose weight reported that they did indeed lose weight. This is a high success rate in an area where success rates are usually low. Since 90 percent of our survey respondents are over the age of fifty, the data show that WBV can be effective for weight loss with older people. Our research is in line with other research showing modest but long-term weight loss with WBV.

Looking fit and trim is great, but there are many important health benefits to losing weight as well. Weight gain and obesity are major health risks and are well known to have a long list of associated diseases. In modern times, with our sedentary lifestyles and easy access to unhealthy but addictive and high-calorie foods, managing our weight is a constant struggle.

The great gift of WBV is that it will not only help you to lose weight, but it will also improve your physical and mental health in many other ways at the same time.

TESTIMONIALS

I've been using WBV and working with Becky for about fifteen years. When I first started, I was forty-seven years old, and I lost thirty pounds in six months. I felt like the Energizer Bunny: I was full of energy, my hay fever and headaches went away, my mood improved, and I became much stronger than I had ever been.

Then I moved out of state, fell out of touch, and stopped using vibration. Gradually, I gained all the weight back plus more, and my health issues came back.

Six years later, I returned and began working with Becky again. The weight is coming off more slowly this time, but I have lost about twenty pounds so far, and as long as I eat well, and vibrate, I can lose weight again.

But mostly, thank God for Becky's incredible ability to help me with my health issues! Over the years, with the help of WBV and Becky's "magic" homeopathic remedies, she has helped me with so many debilitating health concerns: joint pain, weakness, dizziness, nausea, headaches, skin rashes, hot flashes and night sweats, fatigue, wheezing, anxiety, depression, and grief after the deaths of multiple family members and friends.

Today, I am proud to say, I am strong and healthy, working and enjoying my life, calmer and more balanced than ever. Thank you, Becky.

—*Doreen Hadge, age 62*

I am thrilled with my vibration machine. Combining vibration with diet changes and a *Candida* yeast program, I have lost forty pounds in six months—after many years of trying to lose weight with little success. My legs are no

How Whole Body Vibration Helps You Lose Weight

♦ WBV can be an intense workout, and, like any workout, this will increase your metabolic rate so that you burn more calories and lose weight more easily—and the time required to achieve the same results as with traditional exercise forms is much less. Remember: ten minutes of WBV equals one hour of conventional weight training.

♦ The workout will build lean muscle mass that will continue to burn more calories all day long. Lean muscle mass can account for 60 percent of your energy and calorie expenditure while at rest.

♦ WBV raises serotonin levels in your brain, which has a powerful antidepressant effect (see also chapter 5). With your mental state happier and calmer, it will be easier for you to eat properly and exercise. Everybody knows they should eat well (probably lesser quantities as well as healthier choices) and exercise more to lose weight; the problem is actually doing it. WBV helps you to be in that calm and relaxed but energized mental state in which you can focus and achieve your goals.

♦ WBV gives you strength (increased muscle power) and energy (see also chapter 6). So, when you do go out to exercise— now more often because you have more energy, and you are in a better emotional and mental state—you will work harder, consequently burning more calories.

♦ WBV lowers cortisol levels.2 Cortisol is a major stress and aging hormone that promotes fat production and storage. Lowering cortisol levels helps promote fat burning and proper fat metabolism.

♦ WBV improves joint health in numerous ways (see chapters 4 and 6) so that you have greater mobility and are able to exercise more.

longer swollen, and I am off my diuretic medication. I also have had high cholesterol my entire adult life (everybody in my family has high cholesterol), and I have been on Lipitor for years. My cholesterol has now dropped eighty points, and I am off Lipitor. My triglycerides were very high (332)—they have dropped over a hundred points to 214. My gas, bloating, and heartburn have disappeared, and my face is clear—the puffiness, poor color, and minor acne is gone.

—Angelica, age 57

Here's a frequently asked question: Will people see my fat jiggle? No, don't worry! On my machines, at least, only your feet will visibly vibrate.

Scientific Research

The early research with animals was very exciting. In a 2007 study of mice that received fifteen minutes of daily vibration for twelve weeks, the mice that got vibration ended up with 27 percent lower amounts of fat, along with corresponding increases in bone density, than the control mice that didn't get any vibration.[3] In the photo from this study, the dark areas are fat, and the mice who

Mice Exposed to Vibration   Normal Mice

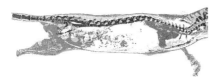 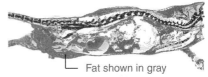

Fat shown in gray

Source: Clinton Rubin; PNAS. Used by permission of Dr. Clinton Rubin.

received vibration are visibly considerably leaner and have less of the dark fat areas.

By 2018, there had been many research studies with people, and the results were less dramatic but still encouraging. In the 2018 systematic review mentioned at the beginning of this chapter, twenty-eight research studies were initially considered for inclusion, ten studies were excluded for various methodological or other reasons, leaving a total of eighteen research studies looking at the effects of WBV for weight loss in adults.[4–21] The combined results of these studies led to the conclusion that "six to twelve weeks of WBVT [Whole Body Vibration Training] in obese individuals generally led to a reduction in fat mass and cardiovascular improvements."[22]

> *The combined results of these studies led to the conclusion that "six to twelve weeks of WBVT in obese individuals generally led to a reduction in fat mass and cardiovascular improvements."*

Eight studies in the review reported a body weight decrease from 5 to 10 percent,[23–29] with one twenty-four-week study showing continued weight loss. That long-term study, a 2010 study of sixty-one overweight and obese adults, saw significant weight loss with a combination of WBV and diet, with the best long-term results obtained for those participants who combined WBV with aerobic exercise and diet. Their conclusions were that

> combining either aerobic exercise or WBV training with caloric restrictions can help to achieve a sustained

long-term weight loss of 5–10%. WBV training may have the potential to reduce VAT [visceral adipose tissue; i.e., fat] more than aerobic exercise in obese adults. . . . Only Fitness and Vibration (participants) managed to maintain a weight loss of 5% or more in the long term.[30]

Fat mass reductions of 2 to 6 percent were seen in seven of the studies[31–37] in that same 2018 review, including in some of the studies where there was no weight change reported. And the weight loss was due to a loss of fat, not lean muscle mass; no studies reported a loss in lean muscle mass, and one study reported an increase in lean muscle mass.[38] Leg muscle strength improved by 8 to 18 percent in four of the eighteen studies.

Twelve of the eighteen studies also looked at arterial and cardiovascular health. Ten studies reported improvements in various measurements of arterial stiffness, with five studies reporting large decreases in blood pressure.[39–43] One study[44] reported a reduction in LDL cholesterol and triglyceride concentrations in the blood.

Additional benefits found included a decline in falling,[45] an increase in oxygen uptake,[46] and an increase in resting energy expenditure,[47] meaning one would be burning fat more efficiently all day.

Hormone Changes

This same review of obesity also included one study[48] that reported a large decrease in fasting insulin levels, which is an indication of improving insulin and glucose metabolism, lowering the risk of insulin resistance, prediabetic and diabetic conditions, high blood sugar levels, and hyperglycemia.

Leptin levels and adiponectin levels also became more balanced. Leptin levels, which are involved in appetite regulation and thermogenesis (heat production) and are typically elevated in obese people, decreased. Adiponectin, another hormone that helps control glucose regulation and fatty acid oxidation and is generally depressed in obese patients, increased.

In 2017, there was great excitement when a researcher at the Medical College of Georgia in Augusta showed that inflammation markers were significantly reduced in type 2 diabetic mice.[49] McGee's results confirmed similar results in an earlier study.[50] *Science* magazine, one of the most highly respected scientific journals in the country, greeted the new research with a hopeful article reporting that "whole-body vibration provides similar metabolic benefits as walking on a treadmill, suggesting it may be useful for treating obesity and Type II diabetes."[51]

Risks and How to Avoid Them

With this group of people, there were few reports of adverse effects with the vibration; a few cases of lower leg phlebitis (inflammation of a vein), a few of mild knee pain, and a couple of reports of back pain. However, the majority of the studies in this review did not include participants who had other health conditions besides obesity (only one included type 2 diabetics, one had fibromyalgia patients, and two included participants with systolic blood pressure higher than 120mmHg). The average age was twenty to fifty-nine years old.

With an older population, and when there are other health conditions, as is often the case especially with older people, researchers may find it more difficult to achieve the same results, and more attention would likely be needed in the area of safety. Some of the studies included in this review used quite powerful machines with amplitudes of 2–5 mm and g-forces up to 21 g. I would not recommend such intense powerful vibration for more vulnerable populations. (Before beginning a WBV program, be sure to check the contraindications on pages 128–131.)

Most research on weight loss with WBV puts a lot of emphasis on the exercise aspect. Virtually all the studies in the 2018 review discussed earlier had participants performing a series of exercises while vibrating. While exercise is an essential part of health and long-term weight control, my experience and research indicate that it is better to begin a WBV program with a very small amount of vibration and build up; it is not necessary to be exercising on the vibration plate, especially in the beginning. I believe that a slow start yields better results because WBV has so many powerful effects, especially on the brain (see chapter 5).

When you are in pain, exhausted, or unmotivated, it is fine to begin by simply standing on the plate. The vibration will flow through your body and mind, helping to reduce your pain and inflammation (chapter 4), improve mood and focus (chapter 5), and improve energy and strength (chapters 1 and 6). When you feel better, it will be easy to add in a more rigorous exercise plan. In Vibrant Health's 2019 survey of our customers (see appendix), 64 percent of the respondents reported that they followed my recommendation to start slowly, and 54 percent said that this was important for their success.

TESTIMONIAL

Theresa Wright participated in a WBV class with the author using a gentle vibration machine of a type similar to that used in Vibrant Health's 2019 survey. The class met once a week for six weeks. Each participant was given one minute of vibration during the first session, and each succeeding week the amount was increased by one minute (class was still held only once per week, so that means she got a total of one minute of WBV the first week, two minutes the second week, etc.). Participants began to use exercise positions in the third week. For the first two weeks, they only stood on the plate.

> I experienced an immediate response to my first whole body vibration session. In the first class, we were each allowed one minute of WBV. Standing on the machine, I felt a powerful soothing sensation in my body. Following the first class, I also felt more energetic. Within two days, I felt more relaxed than before, handled stress better, and my energy level was growing.
>
> Five days after the first session, I experienced a day of super high energy, something I haven't felt for many years. This was the energy level I had had most of my life but that had been gone for several years. Great stamina was back, and cleaning chores were enjoyable and easy. Spending long hours at the computer at my last job before I retired left me hating to use my home computer. Now suddenly that disappeared, and I once again enjoyed using the com-

puter. I couldn't believe how dramatically I was responding to the WBV.

Then there is the weight issue. By combining a healthy diet, natural supplements, exercise, and whole body vibration, I lost nine pounds in six weeks. Having tried to lose weight many times without success, I am sure the whole body vibration helped to make the difference. My scale has blessed me with a number I haven't seen in years.

—*Teresa, early 60s*

Vibrant Health's WBV Research

Regarding weight loss, our 2019 Vibrant Health survey results are similar to the published research discussed above, except our participants' average ages are considerably higher. In our survey of Vibrant Health customers, 50 percent of those who wanted to lose weight did lose, with 24 percent of this group losing one to ten pounds, 10 percent losing ten to twenty pounds, 5 percent losing twenty to thirty pounds, and 10 percent losing more than thirty pounds. Since our customers were mostly not obese, just mildly to moderately overweight, this weight loss is quite significant. An average weight loss of about fifteen pounds, for an estimated average weight person of 150 pounds, would be a 10 percent weight loss; and as this survey covered two years, this weight loss was well maintained.

Of people using Vibrant Health machines, 50 percent of those who wanted to lose weight did lose, sometimes more than thirty pounds.

Most of the participants in Vibrant Health's study did not change their diets, which made it easier to see the effect of the WBV, as we could eliminate diet changes as the cause of their weight loss.

Most of our survey respondents were already on some version of a low carbohydrate diet, and they continued this eating pattern as they added WBV. Low carb diets have been found to be successful at helping people lose weight and improve health. There are many different types of low carb diets: the Zone Diet, the South Beach Diet, the Atkins diet, the Caveman Diet, the ketogenic diet, a *Candida* diet (see more at the end of chapter about this diet), and more. They are variants on a theme, each with particular advantages for different situations but all good for blasting through a weight plateau.

Combining WBV, Aerobic Exercise, and Diet

While WBV is good exercise in many ways, and even has some cardiovascular benefits, it is not an intense aerobic workout. Aerobic exercise has additional benefits to your health, especially for the cardiovascular and respiratory systems, and additional exercise will help you lose weight, too!

There are many diet approaches and exercise methods; the trick is to find what works for you—a diet and exercise program that is effective for you and that you enjoy and can stick with.

"Interval training" is a relatively new method of exercising: high intensity training for short bursts, alternating with short rest periods. With this method, it has been shown that you can cut your total time spent exercising and get the benefits of a much longer workout, including strength and increased metabolism, which helps with weight loss.

You can even do interval training with your WBV workout to maximize your WBV training (you should still add in aerobic exercise). The preprogrammed settings on a Vibrant Health WBV machine include ten-minute routines with automatic time and frequency changes to give you interval training.

Troubleshooting

While I have seen excellent results with many clients (and myself: I once weighed two hundred pounds but have now been 125 pounds for many years), there can be other issues that need to be addressed. If you are not losing weight and inches while using WBV, aerobically exercising, and eating a healthy, low carb diet, possible reasons include:

1. Too much vibration too soon: Vibration has very powerful effects on every part of your body, stimulating every system to work harder, so it can be stressful for you, even while helping you heal and achieve greater health. Too much vibration too soon can stress your body, leading to a temporary increase in inflammation that can cause any health issue to worsen.

Though it is hard to believe, the first thing to try if you are not seeing weight loss is to vibrate less. Everybody wants to vibrate more, thinking more exercise will help. But in this case, because the total effect of WBV is so great, less is more. I see the best results with my clients when we start with one minute and increase slowly.

2. Gut Dysbiosis: Gut dysbiosis is an imbalance of the micro-organisms within our intestines.[52] These microorganisms consist of various strains of bacteria, fungi, and protozoa. Collectively, these microorganisms are known as gut flora. They are essential for digestion and immune functioning, but when the balance is upset, it can result in many digestive and other systemic health issues.

A particularly common issue is an overgrowth of *Candida* yeast. *Candida* can cause gas, bloating, IBS, constipation, diarrhea, and water retention, as well as sugar and carbohydrate cravings and many other symptoms. (See additional research studies for further information, including extensive lists of other symptoms yeast overgrowth can cause.) Used properly, WBV will help to eliminate yeast and balance the gut flora[53] because WBV is such a powerful health-enhancing system. The more you strengthen your overall health, which is linked to your immune system, the less yeast will be able to survive. But because WBV is also a powerful detoxification system, too much WBV can temporarily weaken your immune system, leading to yeast levels increasing, along with the associated symptoms.

As millions of people have high levels of *Candida,* a program to eliminate and control this gut dysbiosis, along with your WBV program, can be extremely helpful—within a week of starting a diet and program specifically designed to eliminate *Candida* yeast, many people will often see dramatic changes. *Candida* yeast overgrowth is an epidemic—some estimates are as high as 80 percent of the people in the US having more *Candida* yeast in their body than they should—so this is an excellent diet to try.

Exactly how much WBV a person will be able to tolerate without aggravating their symptoms varies greatly depending on their overall state of health. If you are still having difficulty, working with a qualified health professional is recommended.

WBV can also help with constipation directly—perhaps by stimulating the abdominal and pelvic muscles.

> I'm fifty-eight and have Epstein Barr and interstitial cystitis. I use my machine fifteen minutes a day, and it makes me feel great—no matter what my symptoms. It relieves my constipation in fifteen minutes and gives me energy! Thank you, Becky!
>
> —Lindsey, age 58

3. Hormonal and metabolic imbalances: If you have eliminated the first two causes for not losing weight, you may have hormonal and/or metabolic imbalances. There are numerous hormonal and metabolic issues that can make it difficult to lose weight. Sometimes you can reset your metabolic and hormonal systems with a stringent diet such as the ketogenic diet. Even more drastically, the "Fast Mimicking Diet" has been shown to stimulate stem cells and bring rapid and dramatic health benefits.

Please consult a qualified health professional to address these issues and continue with your WBV program.

CHAPTER 3

Increasing Bone Density

Building Bone Safely and Naturally

Extensive research over the last forty years has shown that WBV safely promotes and increases bone density, more so than conventional exercise, which has long been understood to be important for healthy bone development. Originally developed for space travelers, who lose bone density at a rate of up to one hundred times faster than a normal person on earth,[1] this breakthrough is of critical importance to postmenopausal women in developed countries, who are experiencing epidemic levels of bone loss. Add to this scenario the very real dangers associated with bone-density drugs, and you have a lifesaving technology that has spurred hundreds of studies and interest all over the world.

Research results with animals and younger, healthy people have been dramatic. The development and use of vibration in the 1970s allowed Russian cosmonauts to be in space twice as long as their nonvibrating American counterparts (approximately two hundred days versus one hundred days). In 2013, a NASA website cited the effects of vibration on turkeys, sheep, and rats as "profound . . . promoting near-normal rates of bone formation"[2] under laboratory conditions simulating the zero gravity conditions of space flight. In other research, Dr. Clinton Rubin, director of the Center for Biotechnology at the State University of New York at Stony Brook, reported increasing the bone density in mice nearly 30 percent with vibration for fifteen minutes a day for fifteen weeks.[3] And a research study with younger, well-trained cyclists showed an increase in bone density of 1.6 percent in just ten weeks.[4]

The results with postmenopausal women have been less clear. While some studies have concluded WBV can help increase bone density,[5, 6] others have found that it failed to increase bone density.[7–9] The research has centered on the different parameters of WBV, such as the frequency, amplitude, and g-force, trying to find the best combination for effective bone building.

The most recent (2018) systematic review and meta-analysis of the subject, focusing on ten clinical trials, concluded that "WBV is an effective method to improve lumbar spine BMD in postmenopausal and older women and to enhance femoral neck BMD in postmenopausal women younger than 65 years."[10, 11] They further conclude that to achieve the best results, the vibration frequency should be at least 20 Hz, and the amplitude and g-force should be at least 5 mm and 8 gs, and it needs to be used over a long period of time (more than 108 sessions). (These g-force numbers are confusing and misleading, however, due to changing methods of calculation—which has led to a doubling of the reported g-force in many cases. Please see chapter 8 for a more detailed explanation of this issue.)

While overall this study is encouraging, a critical missing element in the studies with older people is comprehensive nutritional supplementation, and this is also skewing the results. I pointed this out in my first book on WBV published in 2013, and unfortunately this remains the case today. Studies on bone density typically provide participants with, at most, calcium, magnesium, and vitamin D, but bone building is a complex process requiring more than a dozen critical nutrients, and older people often have decreased nutrient intake and absorption.

The studies with animals and younger people demonstrate clearly that WBV does stimulate bone to increase its density, but building bone involves the healthy functioning of many different systems. As people age, many systems in their bodies do not work as well, so just providing the signal to build bone may not be sufficient intervention.

Vibrant Health's 2019 Survey Research Results

Vibrant Health recently completed a survey of our customers using the Vibrant Health Power 1000 vibration machine. This machine has a lower amplitude and g-force than recommended in the review study discussed above, but our results are similar if not better. In our survey, 40 percent of respondents, 88 percent of whom were between the ages of fifty and eighty, either increased their bone density or did not lose bone density. Those who reported increasing the most were below the age of sixty-five. The vast majority of Vibrant Health's customers are also health conscious, eating an

In our survey, 40 percent of respondents, 88 percent of whom were between the ages of fifty and eighty, either increased their bone density or did not lose bone density.

excellent diet, and taking natural supplements—all of which will help the body build bone.

Despite their healthy lifestyles, many of Vibrant Health's customers had still developed osteopenia or osteoporosis, and almost all were concerned about bone density. Unfortunately, our two-year study did not cover a long enough time period to get a full picture of bone changes, as people at risk of osteoporosis usually get a bone-density scan every three years. Thus, many people could not answer our questions about bone-density. With a longer study possibly our results might be even better.

There were numerous reports of increasing bone density, and we are using a machine and system that brings much better overall results. Our results for strength, energy, pain reduction, mood, and sleep are much better than reported in other research, and our bone-density results appear to be similar. So why not get all the possible benefits?

When you are trying to improve any one part of the body, it is wise to look at the body as a whole, not to sacrifice one part for another. The best way to help any one part will be to help the entire body to operate at its best, because the body and mind together is a complex and complete organism with an ability to heal itself. Optimize your own body's ability to heal itself; give it gentle and loving care, and it will work to heal all the myriad factors involved in running and maintaining itself.

The story of a client several years ago who was using a similar vibration machine to the Power 1000 shows how successful this gentler vibration can be. Mary Onorato, a seventy-year-old woman whose doctor told her that going over a bump in the road or coughing too hard could cause a fracture in her vertebrae because her bone-density test put her in the category of "extremely severe" bone-density loss, experienced a complete reversal of bone loss in two and a half years—to where she ended up with the "bones of a healthy young woman." (See pages 43–45 for more details on Mary's remarkable reversal of osteoporosis.)

How WBV Increases Bone Density

Research by Dr. Rubin, through his work with Marodyne Medical and the LivMD low-intensity vibration device, has shown in studies with animals that small (low amplitude), high-frequency signals can cause bone to grow, a sort of buzz or vibration received from muscle attachments to bone. High-impact signals are not necessary for bone growth, as was once thought. In other words, while the impact of a person's foot against the ground may signal bone to grow, the quivering of muscle fibers against bone as the muscle fibers contract during exercise is also an important signal to your bones to increase bone density.

But, when Dr. Rubin and others tried to replicate his results with people, they were not successful.[12, 13] This may be because while very

To effectively build bone, the WBV must be strong enough to transmit vibration throughout your entire body. Then, just standing on a vibrating plate will cause all muscle fibers to involuntarily contract and release twenty to fifty times per second.

low-intensity vibration will easily transmit through the whole body of a mouse or other small animal, it will not transmit through the whole body of a person standing on the plate. This can easily be understood and experienced by anyone standing on one of these very low-intensity vibration plates— you will feel the physical vibration in your feet and maybe lower legs, but not above your knees.

To effectively build bone, the WBV must be strong enough to transmit vibration throughout your entire body, causing all muscle fibers to involuntarily contract and release twenty to fifty times per second. The Power 1000 machine is strong enough to do this; standing upright on this machine, you will feel the vibration transmitting through your whole body and up into your head— you can feel your muscles quivering from head to toe, and many people comment on the sensations of different parts of their face vibrating.

TESTIMONIALS

After a year of using the vibration machine, my bone density increased by 6 percent in both my hip and spine.

When I reported the results to a doctor in my family, he called it a massive increase in the world of bone density.

—*Diane Warshovsky, age 68*

I've been using the BV1000 vibration machine since I was seventy-two years old. I had been diagnosed with osteoporosis many years earlier when I was in my forties. I have never taken any osteoporosis drugs, but I have been taking a lot of natural supplements for many years. I am now in my mid-seventies, and, according to a recent bone-density test, I have the bones of a healthy forty-year-old. The technician who read my results just about fell on the floor! Based on my bone-density test, she was sure I couldn't be older than sixty-five.

—*Anna Wall, mid-70s*

My latest DEXA scan showed no bone loss—for the first time in ten years! My osteoporosis specialist was delighted and said I could stop taking my bone-density medication. I am thrilled to be off these meds, and the shaking seems to help with depression. I have been vibrating for ten minutes every few days, on the machine Becky recommended for me, for the last two years.

—*Barbara Jordan, age 63*

I am delighted with my WBV machine. When I had my annual checkup a few months ago, the bone density in my lumbar spine and both hips had improved, after four years of steadily decreasing bone density.

Many thanks.

—*Dana, age 63*

(**Note:** Dana is using the Vibrant Health Gentle 500 machine, which is not the machine I would usually recommend for building bone. But, if

there are other serious health issues, it is sometimes better to start with
the gentler machine and work up to using the Vibrant Health Power 1000
machine. In this case, Dana is still successfully slowly building bone, even
using the gentle machine!)

There has been some debate about the best positions and types
of exercise to use on a vibration plate to maximize bone building.
Just standing straight transmits the vibration into your upper torso,
head, and neck, which is effective for increasing bone density in
your spine, hips, and legs—some of the most critical areas. Exercising in a static (stationary) or kinetic (movement) position has
been tried to help get vibration into bones where the position of the
bone is horizontal to the vertical line of the body, such as the femoral neck. At this point, whether static or kinetic exercises are best
is not clear.[14, 15] To impact the arms, hands, wrists, and shoulders,
it is important to use positions where your hands are directly on
the vibrating plate, such as a push-up, which will activate muscles
attached to these bones.

It is clear that longer sessions of WBV (at least ten minutes) are
more effective and that building bone is a slow process—at least
108 sessions are required (at a rate of two to seven times weekly).
Even under the best of circumstances (that is, using WBV daily),
one might see a small increase in bone density after three and a half
months, but most studies run six to nine months.

A mid-range smooth vibration can be effective for increasing
bone density; Vibrant Health's survey research study has shown this.
So, while some other research recommends high intensity vibration
machines, I cannot agree. Larger more powerful machines are often

too stressful for the body and mind to promote optimal healing (see also chapters 4 and 5).

Bone-Density Drugs

Poor nutrition, a lack of exercise, a lack of vitamin D,[iii] and the use of numerous drugs that inhibit proper digestion and assimilations of nutrients and/or bone development have combined to create an epidemic of weak and brittle bones. Statistically, in the US, one third of women and one sixth of men will now experience a hip-bone fracture at some point in their lifetime, and these types of fractures often result in death or permanent loss of independence and mobility.

In response, the pharmaceutical industry and Western medicine have developed, and heavily promoted, a class of drugs called bisphosphonates. These include all those drugs advertised by movie stars and celebrities on TV: Fosamax, Actonel, Boniva, and Reclast. These drugs do result in tests showing an increase in bone density—but beware! They achieve an increase in bone density by halting your body's natural ability to reabsorb old and damaged bone. The result is more bone, but it is weak, old, and fragile bone. The situation is most acute in the jawbone, where increased blood flow supports the extra bone repair that is normal in that area.

This causes a concentration of the drugs and their effects and has led to a surge in cases of a horrifying condition called osteonecrosis (bone death) of the jaw (ONJ). Unfortunately, this process

---

[iii]Sunshine causes the body to create vitamin D, but sun exposure is avoided by or not available to many people for much of the year.

of bone death and rot is usually painless and hidden, so it goes unnoticed for years, until the person goes to the dentist for a surgical procedure. Then, with exposure to the bacteria in the mouth and the increased demand for healing, a major disaster follows, with permanent, untreatable pain; disfigurement; and great difficulty eating.

Fosamax, Actonel, Boniva, and Reclast . . . achieve an increase in bone density by halting your body's natural ability to reabsorb old and damaged bone.

Another area in which this drug-induced bone weakness is showing up is in a bizarre type of severe thigh-bone fracture that happens without any unusual stress on the bone. People who have been taking bisphosphonates for five or more years (though occasionally this problem shows up within months) are ending up in emergency rooms with cross-transverse compound fractures of the femur bone from merely standing up or walking. These are still very rare occurrences, but they may be about to become more common as hundreds of thousands of Americans who have been on these drugs for many years reach the critical time period.

Normal Bone Growth

Healthy bone formation and growth is a complex process involving numerous systems in the body, including bone building and remodeling cells within the bone itself, digestion, hormones, the liver and kidneys, and the presence in plentiful amounts of more than a dozen minerals and vitamins. An excellent book in which this process is extensively researched and clearly detailed is *Your Bones: How You Can Prevent Osteoporosis and Have Strong Bones for Life—Naturally,* by Lara Pizzorno, the editor and author of numerous natural health publications and books.

Excellent nutrition and a healthy digestive system that is able to extract and absorb all the necessary nutrients are of critical importance to building bone. In addition to calcium, magnesium, and phosphorus, it is also necessary to have available the minerals strontium, boron, zinc, manganese, copper, silicon, molybdenum, and selenium and vitamins A, C, D, K_1, K_2, B_6, B_{12}, folate, and riboflavin.

Luckily, a healthy diet for building bone is the same diet that is healthy for every other part of you. A primarily plant-based, whole-foods diet with small amounts of animal products, if desired, will make an enormous difference to your health. This will supply the nutrients that every part of your body requires to function, and all the systems in your body will work better. In deep and scary contrast is the average American diet with its heavy load of junk and fast food and mind-bogglingly tiny portions of fruits and vegetables. The second National Health and Nutrition Examination survey found that only 27 percent of Americans are eating three servings of fruits and vegetables per day, but this included potatoes, most of which were eaten as french fries and chips! Chips and fries don't count as part of a healthy diet.

Within our bones, one type of specialized bone cell, called an osteoclast, breaks down old and worn-out bone. Another type of bone cell, called an osteoblast, is a bone-forming cell that pulls calcium, magnesium, and phosphorus from the blood to build new bone. Without the osteoclasts, damaged bone builds up, leading to weak bone; without healthy osteoblast activity, new bone will not be formed. Bisphosphonate drugs increase total bone density by killing the osteoclast cells; the result is weak and diseased bone. WBV will signal your body to increase bone density without interfering with the removal of old and weak bone.

Older People and Bone Growth

As people age, critical systems for bone building may not function as well: digestion and assimilation of nutrients may be poor; hormonal changes decrease bone building (especially in women); and older people are often taking drugs that interfere in some way with the process of building bone. For example, people with low stomach acid do not digest and absorb many nutrients (including only about 4 percent of the most commonly used form of calcium supplement, calcium carbonate), and studies have shown that about 40 percent of postmenopausal women are severely deficient in stomach acid.

Even worse, many of these people will end up further compounding the problem by taking antacids and other drugs (over-the-counter or prescription) for "acid reflux," when in fact the problem is poor digestion due to too little acid, not enough enzymes, or *Candida* yeast overgrowth—all of which could be resolved easily and quickly with natural treatments.

Western medicine is notoriously poor in its understanding and approach to nutrition. So WBV bone-density studies do not provide the full range of necessary nutrients to participants. But you cannot build a house with only lumber and nails. You also need nail guns, workers, screws, measuring tools, siding, sheetrock, windows, doors, etc. It is the same with building bone—there are many critical elements, and nothing at all can happen without them. The vibration supplies the signal, something like a foreman yelling, "Let's go," and the calcium and magnesium could be the lumber, but where are the workers, nails, nail guns, etc.? What you end up with is a lot of lumber lying on the ground, and a foreman yelling, "Let's go! Let's go!"

Nutritional Supplements

Healthy, whole-food choices are important, but the truth is that even with excellent food choices, because our food supply is so compromised by poor soils, overuse of nitrogen fertilizers, early picking, and long shipping and storage times, not to mention food processing that destroys the remaining nutrients, it can be very difficult to get enough nutrition to reverse existing health issues. For this reason, I generally recommend taking high-quality nutritional supplements along with eating a healthy diet. An excellent comprehensive mineral and vitamin bone-building supplement, providing more than two dozen nutrients important for bone growth, is a product called Pro-Bono, made by Ortho Molecular Products. Another product I can recommend is the plant-based supplement called Bone Renewal made by Pure Synergy.

Documented Case Study

Mary Onorato has the most dramatic and well-documented case among my clients. Over the course of five years, she had four

DEXA exams (the gold standard of bone-density testing) to track her extremely severe osteoporosis, all at the same hospital and with the same equipment. After two years of slowly declining bone density, despite a strict routine of comprehensive mineral and vitamin supplementation and regular weightlifting and walking, she found me and began WBV in April 2004. From then on, her DEXA scans began a sudden and dramatic turnaround (see graph below).

Mary never took any bone-building prescription drugs and had stopped the weightlifting and walking several months prior to meeting me and beginning WBV, but she continued with her nutritional supplements. The only change in her program once she met me was the addition of WBV. For the first year, Mary used a powerful double-motor vibration machine, the same one I was using early on. During this period, Mary's bone density slowly increased. After the

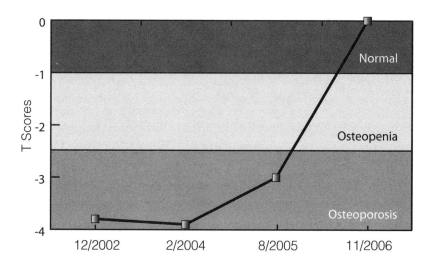

Mary Onorato's Lumbar Spine Bone Density

first year and a half, in October 2005, she switched (along with me) to a gentler machine with a vibration similar to the Power 1000 machine. Mary's bone density then actually began to increase more quickly (see graph). Both types of WBV were clearly providing a signal to her body to build bone, but it appears that the overall healthier signal of the gentler machine helped her body to respond more strongly to that signal.

Note: Mary Onorato's results are not typical, but they are well documented and clearly show the effects of WBV. Most of my other postmenopausal clients with osteopenia or osteoporosis build bone at a slower rate, usually 2 to 6 percent over six months. These results are from my clients' bone-density studies as reported to me; they are not part of a published study. They are, however, significantly better than published studies of WBV's effect on bone building in postmenopausal women.

CHAPTER 4

Pain and Inflammation

If you are a senior, the chances are high that you have got some chronic aches and pains. Almost everybody will have some osteoarthritis by the age of sixty. Our feet hurt, our knees hurt, our backs and shoulders are causing trouble—and that's just the joints! There are stomach and digestive problems, heart and kidney issues, and the list goes on. . . .

These aches and pains are not a death sentence; they are your body saying, "Wake up, help me!" Pay attention, and give yourself love and care, like you would for a child crying in pain.

Pain and high inflammation levels have been linked to almost all chronic health problems, so lowering pain and inflammation levels is the goal of many health interventions. This goal can be accomplished directly with medications or natural products and with therapies such as yoga and meditation, which calm and de-stress your mind and body.[1]

Whole body vibration, when used properly, can also dramatically decrease pain and inflammation, and in the best possible way—by helping your body and mind to heal themselves.

Whole body vibration, when used properly, can also dramatically decrease pain and inflammation, and in the best possible way—by helping your body and mind to heal themselves.

Scientific Research on WBV and Pain

Research has shown clear evidence that some types of pain, such as chronic lower back pain, decrease with WBV.[2–5] Lower back pain is often due to chronic muscle and connective tissue pain, and the powerful effect of WBV relaxing and strengthening muscles is thought to help with this type of discomfort.[6] Other WBV studies have shown improvements in muscle pain,[7] fibromyalgia,[8] and knee pain from osteoarthritis.[9–11]

But for some types of pain—for example, knee osteoarthritis (KOA)—the results have not been clear. While some studies with older people conclude that WBV improves knee osteoarthritis pain,[12–14] others conclude that it doesn't.[15–17] One systematic review and meta-analysis (these terms describe different types of studies; they are often combined, but they are not the same[iv]) research study[18] based on five clinical trials on this subject concluded that the combined

---

[iv]Systematic review research studies consider all the available research studies on a subject and choose those that meet the highest standards of research (peer reviewed, randomized, double-blinded clinical trials with proper controls, English language, and other statistical factors). Meta-analysis refers to statistical analysis of the results of all the included studies together. Most, but not all, systematic reviews use meta-analysis methods to analyze the pooled data. In this particular study, out of eighty-three studies originally identified, five met all the requirements and were included for analysis. Systematic reviews are considered the highest quality evidence on a research subject. But, while these studies are thought to be the most reliable and free of bias, the effect of money is not taken into account. Scientific research in this country and elsewhere is heavily influenced by money. The type of clinical research trial that meets the highest requirements takes a great deal of money, effectively silencing many good ideas and people.

data showed statistically significant improvement in knee pain and function. But, individually, only two of the five studies in that meta-analysis concluded that knee pain was reduced.[19] Another systematic review concluded that KOA pain does not decrease with WBV.[20]

Research on WBV and Inflammation

Meanwhile, several studies have shown decreased inflammation with WBV by looking at levels of specific molecules in the body that are associated with inflammation (inflammation markers). One of the knee osteoarthritis studies discussed earlier, which did report decreased pain, also showed reduced inflammatory markers.[21] Another recent study showed lowered inflammation with WBV use in patients with fibromyalgia.[22]

As mentioned in chapter 2, there was also great excitement in 2017 when researchers showed that inflammation markers were significantly reduced in type 2 diabetic mice.[23]

However, these indications that inflammation can be reduced with WBV have not seemed to pan out into good results with pain research. There are currently few studies on WBV's effects on inflammation in people. As more studies are done on inflammation in people, I suspect that, as with pain research, researchers will have difficulty consistently reproducing the encouraging preliminary results.

What accounts for the conflicting results?

The answer lies in how and what type of WBV is used, especially with more fragile populations, such as older people and those with health issues.

Vibrant Health's WBV Survey Pain Results

In our 2019 WBV survey (see appendix), we asked the thirty-nine respondents who had pain when they first began their WBV program to rate their overall pain levels before and after beginning WBV on a scale from 1 to 10, where 1 equaled "no pain" and 10 equaled "extreme pain." The study covered a two-year period with respondents having used WBV from one month to two years. For all respondents who initially reported pain (88 percent of whom were fifty to eighty years of age), there was an average 31 percent drop in pain levels. Before beginning WBV, the average reported pain level was 5.2; after WBV, the average pain level was 3.6. While not every person's pain improved with WBV, numerous people reported rapid and dramatic drops in their pain levels.

The reductions seen in pain levels are particularly striking given that after beginning WBV, 22 percent of respondents stopped using their pain medications, reduced the amount, or changed to less powerful medications.

Rapid Relief for Many Types of Pain

In Vibrant Health's survey, numerous different types of pain improved, most notably for joints throughout the body, back pain, muscle pain, nerve pain, and headaches.

Of those participants reporting joint pain improvement, 75 percent had knee pain, 33 percent hip pain, 42 percent shoulder pain, 25 percent elbow pain, 25 percent wrists/hands pain, and 17 percent ankles/feet pain. Many had multiple types of pain and often reported improvements in different areas simultaneously. This sort of systemic effect will be discussed in further detail later.

We asked respondents whose pain improved (74 percent) for more details.

In our survey, 74 percent of those in pain saw a 52 percent drop in their pain levels.

They reported an average decrease in pain of over 52 percent for many different types and locations of joint, muscle, lower back, and nerve pains. Other researchers have also seen reductions in pain for muscle,[24] knee,[25] and lower back pain.[26]

Rapid Pain Reduction

- Muscle pain: 20 percent of respondents reported an improvement in muscle pain after only one WBV session; 80 percent reported improvements after a few WBV sessions.

- Joint pain: 9 percent of respondents reported improvements after one WBV session; 82 percent reported improvements within two weeks.

- Back pain: 27 percent noticed an improvement immediately; 90 percent by one month.

- Nerve pain: 33 percent noticed improvement after one session; 100 percent within two weeks.

Of thirty-nine respondents with pain initially, only eleven did not report an improvement. Seventy-four percent of all respondents who had pain experienced relief.

Pain levels dropped extremely quickly. Many reported feeling better almost immediately; within weeks, almost everybody was reporting improvements.

Pain levels dropped extremely quickly for muscle, joint, back, and nerve pain. Many survey respondents reported feeling better almost immediately; within several weeks, over 50 percent were reporting improvements.

These very rapid changes, especially improvements immediately after one session or within a few WBV sessions, suggests that it is WBV, not some other unaccounted-for factor, that is responsible for the changes reported.

Why Are Vibrant Health's Results So Much Better Than Other Research Results?

In a nutshell, most researchers are using too much vibration—the intensity of the vibration experience is too great. Many are also using powerful vibration machines that can create a wilder motion and an unsynchronized vibration. This can send a desynchronized message into the brain (see also chapter 5)—the opposite of the calming, de-stressing message that is most effective for healing. These two factors, intensity and quality, are critical; when they are not correct, WBV can create too much stress for the body and mind, leading to poor results.

WBV is much more than just a workout. It affects every part of our bodies, including our brain and nervous system, and as your brain is guiding your internal health and well-being along with the rest of your life, it is critical to use vibration that is calming and synchronizing.

People, including researchers, WBV companies, and consumers, don't realize how powerful WBV really is. WBV was originally developed for Olympic athletes, and it is still best known, marketed, and sold for its intense workout effect. Because of this tunnel-vision bias, where increased muscle strength is the expected and primary goal of WBV, researchers use machines that are too powerful and not carefully designed for the smooth, synchronized vibration that is best for your brain, and they try to do too much WBV too soon.

Some of the conflicting results for pain and inflammation can be explained by looking at which machines were used in the different studies. One of the two studies that saw decreased pain in the systematic review of knee osteoarthritis research discussed above used a Turbosonic vibration machine. This is a very expensive ($10–15K) but completely synchronized type of vibration. In the other study reporting positive results, it is not clear exactly what machine and parameters of vibration were used. It was reported that they used a FitVibe vibration machine at a frequency of 35–40 Hz, but FitVibe only makes machines that go up to 20 Hz. If they were actually giving their study participants 20 Hz vibration, this would lower the amount of vibration significantly and might explain why their results were better. Unfortunately, the study was done in another country, and I could not contact them for clarification.

In contrast, most of the other studies either used machines in which two motors create a powerful vibration, or they used a "pivotal" type of vibration machine—neither of which is ideal (see also chapter 8 for more about different types of machines). Two motors can never be perfectly synchronized, leading to a desynchronizing message going into your nervous system and brain with potentially very negative results. A pivotal vibration machine creates a much wilder motion, with one side of the plate going up while the other goes down—something like having each foot on either end of a see-saw. This pivotal motion is large enough that, unless the machine is a very inexpensive model, it will come with handles and bars on three sides to hold on to. As the goal is to calm the mind and de-stress, being on a plate that feels like you might go flying off it is not ideal.

The other major problem with many research studies is just too much vibration too soon. WBV is waking up and stimulating every neuron, cell, organ, and system in your body, calling on them to work harder. This can lead to many improvements in your health as your body tries to heal itself, but it is also taxing (i.e., stressful) for the body and mind, especially the increased detoxification (see chapter 7). More stress on a person's body and mind than they can handle easily leads to inflammation levels increasing,[27] which will slow down improvement, and it can even cause symptoms to worsen instead of improving.

Earlier studies may have been more successful because they were mostly done on research animals or healthy young people, often athletes. They do not use large, powerful (desynchronizing) machines with little animals (the most common research animal is mice), and healthy young people can tolerate much more vibration—without tipping into an overly stressful zone—than older people can.

On the other end of the spectrum, there have also been quite a few studies with extremely gentle vibration machines, producing only 0.3 gs of force. But these machines were not found to be powerful enough to be effective for increasing bone density in people,[28] and when this area of research didn't pan out, interest in these machines declined.

Vibrant Health machines provide vibration that is a sweet spot between the high and low extremes. They provide a smooth, purely synchronized vibration, with an amplitude, g-force, and frequency range that creates just the right degree of intensity—effective but not too stressful. With a careful program of use, rapid pain relief is the result for most people.

Intensity

The intensity of WBV is based on a combination of factors: the amplitude, frequency, amount of time vibrating per session, and how often sessions were done. In all of the published studies mentioned above, the amplitude and amount of time vibrating per session was greater than I would recommend. They all used high amplitude machines (2–5 mm, 2–15 g-force), except for one study that did not report amplitude (an indication of how little they thought it mattered). Accurately discussing amplitude and g-force is difficult, as there are different methods of calculating these parameters—resulting in a twofold, or more, difference in the reported figures—and no one reports which method they are using.[v] I can say that, in general, I recommend lower amplitudes and g-forces than reported in the study discussed above. See chapter 8 for more information on machine specifications and which machine to use. Though a change of a few millimeters may not seem large on paper, the difference in sensation and results is vast.

The minimum amount of time at the beginning of these studies was usually two to three minutes, progressing gradually over eight to twelve weeks to five to ten minutes. One study started with twenty minutes of vibration per session, though this study also used a much lower frequency of vibration (12–14 Hz) than the others. I recommend only thirty to sixty seconds for the first session, because while some people can tolerate more without a problem, some cannot, and you can always increase the amount of vibration.

Most studies use two to three WBV sessions per week, which is fine, as is increasing one minute per week—but only if the individual can easily tolerate this. WBV should be tailored to the individual, and the intensity only increased as they can tolerate it. "Tolerating" means that all symptoms are either staying the same or improving, as too much stress can show up as a worsening of any health issue— in any part of the body or mind.

---

[v]Amplitude is a critical aspect of vibration; a small change in this number can make a large difference in the experience and results. Amplitude can be measured from a centerline to the greatest height or from peak to peak of displacement (movement)—the second method leading to a number twice as large as the first method (see chapter 9 for diagram). Because people want a high-amplitude, powerful machine, some companies inflate their amplitude numbers by using the peak-to-peak measuring method. Many other companies simply don't post any amplitude measurements on their websites. G-force is calculated using the amplitude, so this practice can lead to deceptive g-force claims as well.

Vibrant Health Recommends a Slow and Careful Approach to WBV

How much WBV (i.e., stress) a person can tolerate depends on the state of that person's health. If your body and/or mind are weakened by age, illness, or any other factor, you will not be able to tolerate as much stress as a healthy young person. Trying to start out with a lot of vibration when you are older is like trying to run a race when you are having trouble walking. Just as you would slowly build up to run a race, you should start slowly with WBV; this may mean very slow.

Even a very small amount of WBV can have a strong positive effect, and too much can be disastrous. So it is wise to start with just a tiny amount (thirty to sixty seconds) at the lowest speed setting on the right type of machine.

Then, notice how you feel over the next twenty-four hours, because if inflammation levels are rising, the effects may not be immediately apparent. If any symptoms or health issues worsen over the following twenty-four hours, it is possible that was too much vibration for you, and I would recommend slowing down. It is, of course, possible that you are worse for some other reason, but with some experimentation you can figure this out.

On the other hand, if you are feeling either the same or better the day after vibration, then you can increase the amount of vibration—*a little bit*. See chapter 9 for detailed plans on how to get started.

In Vibrant Health's WBV survey, one respondent's pain levels suddenly and dramatically increased with vibration—but she had increased too fast and used her machine too soon after surgery—a contraindication (see complete contraindication list on pages 124–127). The first time she used her machine, for two minutes, a tooth that had been bothering her and was already slated for implant surgery, suddenly got worse. She stopped vibrating and had the dental surgery. The surgery was needed regardless and was completely unrelated to the WBV, but it was very painful, she reported to me.

After surgery or any other stressful experience with high pain levels, you need to be careful with WBV. Instead, a couple of days later she tried vibration again; this time for three minutes. Within hours, her tooth pain level jumped from "no pain" to "extreme pain." Her pain was gone again the next day, but pain indicates stress on the body—vibration, which adds more stress, should be used with care and caution.

How Does WBV Lower Pain and Inflammation?

Vibrant Health's survey results show pain levels going down for many joint pains all over the body, and for other types of pain in different areas of the body. These widespread and often simultaneous effects indicate that WBV is working in a systemic way to improve health.

Building muscle strength is a terrific goal for many reasons and is highly protective for long-term joint health, but it is not required for rapid initial pain relief.

Pain commonly begins decreasing with only a few very short vibration sessions, with people who are only standing relaxed on the machine. This is not significant exercise; clearly, increasing muscle strength is not the primary initial requirement for lowering pain. Of course, building muscle strength is a terrific goal for many reasons and is highly protective for long-term joint health, but it is not required for rapid initial pain relief.

There are several possible WBV effects that could contribute to lowered pain and inflammation. WBV increases circulation (as does all exercise), bringing nutrients and oxygen to and removing waste products from all tissues. It also increases detoxification by stimulating the lymphatic system due to muscle fibers tensing and relaxing around the lymphatic vessels at the same rate the machine is vibrating.

However, it is doubtful that these effects could cause the extremely rapid changes that often happen with tiny amounts of vibration, so I believe there must be another effect that could account for such rapid changes. But consider, even a very small amount of WBV is a massive stimulation of the nervous system and brain. Billions of neurons will fire signals into the brain at the same rate the machine is vibrating, so even one minute of vibration can have a large effect on the brain; and our mind, dwelling within our brain, controls our whole body and life.

Even a very small amount of WBV is a massive stimulation of the nervous system and brain. . . . Perhaps WBV's most powerful effect is how it can stimulate and tune [these systems].

Perhaps WBV's most powerful effect is how it can stimulate and tune our nervous system and brain.

TESTIMONIALS

One year ago, according to the medical profession, I needed both shoulders replaced. I was in a great deal of pain for years and was unable to raise my arms to reach anything above my head due to the pain and joint limitations. I had to modify all my exercise and drop cross-country skiing, mountain climbing, and yoga because of the pain and limited use of my shoulders and upper body. Depression from this limiting situation had me crying many days, as exercise and wellness had always been a huge part of my life. The pain was intense, twenty-four hours a day.

After only a few sessions, starting at only one minute the first time and increasing only one minute per session, I noticed I was starting to feel better. At first, I wouldn't tell anyone, because I couldn't believe it! But I continued to improve.

Vibrating, in combination with eating well and an exercise program, has been a huge factor in lessening the twenty-four-hour pain I had in both shoulders. The shoulders still need replacing, but, because the pain is not bothering me, I can postpone the medical procedure.

—*Wendy MacLean, senior citizen*

When I first started working with Becky, about three months ago, I had constant pain in my right hip, right thigh, and both knees. I frequently walked with a limp, and climbing stairs was excruciatingly painful. In the last three months, I have made dramatic improvements. I was able to return to moderate exercising, and I have no pain in my hips or thighs. If anyone had told me that

I could be so much stronger or that my pain could be reduced so much in such a brief period of time, I never would have believed it.

—*Ann MacGibbon, PhD, age 58*

CHAPTER 5

Get Smart and Protect Your Brain

A Wondrous Gift

As a senior, it is more critical than ever to take care of your brain. Your brain guides your life and body; it is the home of your mind and soul; and it is the center of your nervous system, connecting you to everything in the universe and making you a unique being of vast potential. Our brains are highly vulnerable to aging, but they can also be one of our most powerful tools in the quest to stay vibrant and active.

During the first few years of life, your brain is growing rapidly, creating more than one million new neural connections every second. During preschool, your brain increases in mass four-fold; by age six, it has reached around 90 percent of adult volume. But as a senior, your brain has begun to lose mass, as neural cells are dying faster than they are being regenerated. Memory and other cognitive functions begin to decrease, and, for some, the fear of serious brain disorders looms.

Whole body vibration will help your brain stay healthy and vibrant well into old age. Even a small amount of WBV will light up your brain as all your neurons automatically fire, sending signals to your brain at the same rate the machine is vibrating. Whole body vibration is intensive exercise, and the latest research is that nothing helps your brain develop and stay healthy more than exercise. A recent *New York Times* magazine article, "Jogging Your Brain," states,

> For more than a decade, neuroscientists and physiologists have been gathering evidence of the beneficial relationship between exercise and brainpower. But the newest findings make it clear that this isn't just *a* relationship, it is *the* relationship.
>
> Exercise, the latest neuroscience suggests, does more to bolster thinking than thinking does.[1]

Whole body vibration is well accepted as intensive exercise when used for that purpose. Hundreds of research studies, top athletes around the world, and, in fact, anybody who has ever tried working out on a powerful vibration plate with muscles begging for relief can attest to this. Yet, even if you only stand on a vibrating plate, you will be stimulating muscles to contract and neurons to fire twenty to fifty times per second, which adds up to ten to fifteen thousand times in one ten-minute session—massive neurological stimulation. Sending signals around your body and brain is a workout for your neurons,

"Exercise . . . does more to bolster thinking than thinking does."

and just as a workout strengthens your muscles, this neurological workout strengthens and protects your neurons.

With a wide variety of possible positions on the plate and intensities of vibration, WBV can be adapted for all levels of physical ability. This allows almost anybody—from a pro athlete to a wheelchair-bound person; from a busy professional to a depressed, unmotivated low achiever—to experience the neurological and other benefits of exercise.

Your Brain's Complexity

Your brain contains one hundred to two hundred billion neurons (nerve cells). Each neuron connects to up to one thousand other neurons through dendrites (thin nerve-tissue filaments), which make up a branching, treelike structure. These connections between neurons are called synapses, and there are some three hundred trillion synapses in a brain, creating vast networks of interconnected neurons. At each synapse, signals leap across a tiny "synaptic gap" via natural chemicals called neurotransmitters, activating an electrical signal that shoots through the next neuron. The latest research shows that there are one thousand activation sites for these neurotransmitters per synapse.

The result is a brain in which there are more neurons than people on earth, more synapses than stars in our galaxy, and more complexity than in all the computers on earth put together. Stretch out all those dendrites plus axons (the part of the neuron that is like the trunk of a tree with a root system that connects to organs and tissues up to three feet away), and they would reach to the moon and back.

It is this very complexity, especially the number of connections between neurons, that gives us our intelligence. "Thinking" involves neurons sending electrochemical signals across the synaptic gaps, lighting up pathways throughout that vast network of billions of neurons in your brain.

Whole Body Vibration Is a Natural Antidepressant

Two neurotransmitters, serotonin and norepinephrine, have been shown to increase with WBV.[2] Serotonin is an important neurotransmitter in your brain that contributes to sounder sleep and feelings of mastery, pleasure, and relaxation. This is the same neurotransmitter that is targeted by prescription antidepressant drugs such as Prozac and Wellbutrin, as well as many illegal drugs such as marijuana, cocaine, and Ecstasy. While prescription drugs for depression can be valuable for helping to alleviate symptoms, they also have side effects, and they can lead to increasing tolerance and dependence on those drugs. Whole body vibration is a natural, safe, rapid, nonaddictive, and legal way to increase serotonin and norepinephrine.

Whole body vibration is a natural, safe, rapid, nonaddictive, and legal way to increase serotonin and norepinephrine.

Norepinephrine is both a neurotransmitter and a hormone, and low levels of this essential molecule have been linked to depression and low energy. Norepinephrine (along with epinephrine) underlies the fight-or-flight response, giving the body sudden energy in times of stress; it increases the heart rate, triggers the release of glucose from energy stores, increases blood flow to skeletal muscles and oxygen supply to the brain, and it can suppress nerve inflammation.

Studies with rats have shown rapid increases in serotonin levels with WBV,[3] but physical measurements of brain serotonin levels can only be done in animals (as brain tissue samples must be taken). Anecdotal evidence of increased serotonin and norepinephrine levels with WBV is strong. Hundreds of my clients (see also the appendix for Vibrant Health's WBV survey results), and thousands of users around the world, report rapid and dramatic improvements in mood, energy, and sleep within days of beginning vibration. They also report increased motivation, focus, and activity levels—perhaps the reason why Tony Robbins, the well-known motivational speaker, uses vibration machines at his seminars. This is an area of great potential and should be investigated more thoroughly.

Hundreds of my clients report rapid and dramatic improvements in mood, energy, and sleep.

TESTIMONIALS

Since I started vibrating two months ago, I am so much calmer and happier than I was—and sleeping more soundly. My kids say, "Mom, you're definitely less uptight and angry."

—Monica Calzolari

I have become addicted to my vibration plate, even if it's only for a few minutes a day. It's my feel-good therapy—a day without vibrating is like a day without sunshine! It just makes you feel so good.

—*Frankie Boyer, radio personality*

I am happier and have more energy now than I ever did when I was on Prozac.

—*Anonymous*

I feel so relaxed after just a few minutes of vibration, it feels like I've just had acupuncture or just gotten out of a hot tub and had a shot of bourbon. The next day, I have more energy than usual—my exhausted and tough Fridays now feel more like a Monday or Tuesday. My sister-in-law also tried the vibration with me one evening and said she slept better that night than she had in years.

—*Mary Beth Little*

Neurogenesis and Plasticity

Neurogenesis is the creation of new brain cells. This was once thought to happen only before birth, but it is now known that, at a slower pace, neurogenesis does continue throughout life. This neurogenesis allows for brain "plasticity," meaning that it can continue to grow and change throughout life, making new neural connections that allow you not only to learn new skills and knowledge but also to increase your ability to learn, think creatively, and change.

An amazing example of neurogenesis and brain plasticity later in life is a new therapy that has been developed for stroke victims who have been paralyzed. Intensive physical therapy for many hours per day with the paralyzed limb, while the normal arm and hand are immobilized, results in the regeneration of brain matter and physical function for people who have suffered complete paralysis of one arm and hand—even as long as seventeen years after the event.

Exercise triggers neurogenesis by prompting the production of brain-derived neurotropic factor (BDNF), which strengthens cells and axons and the connections among neurons, as well as sparking the formation of new neurons. BDNF is thus a physical mediator for increasing the complexity and strength of the neural network in the part of the brain that reflects intellectual potential.

Research showing this connection between exercise and the brain has primarily been done with aerobic exercise. However, similar neurological and muscular processes are involved with weight-lifting-type exercises, to which WBV is most similar. Perhaps WBV, with its massive neurological stimulation, will eventually be found to stimulate BDNF and brain development even more effectively than other forms of exercise; scientific research in this area is eagerly awaited.

Neurological Diseases

Research using WBV for neurological diseases and conditions has so far been conflicted. While there have been good results for cerebral palsy patients, results from studies on Parkinson's, multiple sclerosis, and stroke patients has been less clear. I believe that a major reason for the consistently good results for CP patients is that the subjects are primarily children (CP is a brain disorder that develops before, during, or shortly after birth), and children respond very well to WBV because of greater neuroplasticity and higher energy. These qualities give children the ability to react positively to nuerological interventions and a greater tolerance for stress.

That children have the energy to rebound from stress more easily means that using more WBV with them will still result in a positive outcome. In the case of seniors, especially if they are also ill, you must use a gentler approach; then excellent results may be obtained—just as I have been able to get excellent results with pain and inflammation in seniors by using the right machine and approach.

Regarding the conflicting results of the impact of WBV on Parkinson's and MS patients, I feel it may have more to do with the kinds of machines and the amount of WBV that was used. I have several patients with Parkinson's, multiple sclerosis, or dementia who have reported significant improvements using my machines, which are gentler and more appropriate for the elderly and/or ill.

Parkinson's

A 2014 systematic review of six research studies on this subject concluded that "the majority of studies seem to suggest a favorable benefit following WBV for mobility and balance, but not when compared to other active intervention or placebo."[4] All the studies saw improvements, with three of the six studies finding a greater improvement in balance or mobility than a placebo or other physical therapy. There was no clear pattern, though, as to why some studies resulted in better outcomes than the others.

However, none of these six studies used the type of machine I recommend, with the very slow start and careful increase method that I recommend. Since a couple of my customers with Parkinson's have reported that WBV with their Vibrant Health machine is helping them, I would like to see studies using this type of vibration and method with Parkinson's and other neurological diseases.

Multiple Sclerosis (MS)

With MS, the situation is similar. While a systematic review in 2012 of WBV and MS found that "some investigations have shown significant improvements of the muscle strength, of the functional mobility, and of the timed get up and go test in patients with MS,"[5] they concluded there were not enough good quality studies to make recommendations as to what type of machine and method of use would reliably lead to benefits. They recommended more research.

A clinical trial in 2018 attempting to clarify the situation studied twenty-one women, ages eighteen to sixty-four, with MS.[6] It is unclear what type of machine they were using. The study reports using a Power Plate: Next Generation vertical vibration machine with a "low amplitude" setting of 3 mm. A 3 mm amplitude is not what I would consider low, so I contacted Power Plate. The representative I spoke to told me that the low amplitude setting on that model would be 1–2 mm. More importantly, they also told me that regardless of whether that model is used on its low or high amplitude setting, it will always be using two motors—it is a double motor machine, the type I most strongly recommend not using because of the possibility of brain desynchronization (see page 85).

In this study, subjects were given shorter vibration sessions than in many studies, only two and a half minutes once a week for five weeks, but it is still more than I recommend. For someone with a significant health issue, I recommend thirty seconds for the first session, repeated up to three times a week, then increasing to one minute three times per week, and so on (see chapter 9 for more detail on my recommended protocols).

The basic rule with vibration and health problems is that the sicker you are, the less vibration you should do.

The study results were not encouraging—they basically saw no improvements. This is not unexpected to me; my experience is that you will not effectively improve brain function using the wrong type of vibration—especially if the brain and body are already stressed, as is the case with illness.

As with many studies, this one ends with the recommendation to do more research, increasing the amount of vibration. My recommendation would also be to do more research, but with *less* vibration and the right type of vibration. Researchers have tried less vibration but not little enough and not on the correct schedule with the correct machines. The best results come with a very small amount of WBV, regularly applied over a long time (weeks to months), building up slowly but with a resting period of a day or two to recover after each small session—all using the best type of vibration.

The basic rule with vibration and health problems is that the sicker you are, the less vibration you should do. It's really hard to follow that rule; the tendency and desire is always to do more, but use that energy to make sure you are also getting the proper nutrition and supplements to support healing in your body and mind, and add in other therapies, such as exercise and energy medicine.

Stroke

The situation is similar with stroke research. A large 2019 systematic review,[7] including a total of forty-six research studies, looked at the effects of WBV on gait and movement. Seven of the studies were on stroke patients. Two of these seven reported improvements in walking speed and quality after WBV. The review's overall conclusion for stroke patients was that WBV is effective for improving walking performance, but only two out of the seven stroke studies individually reported benefits.

Healing the brain and body from any significant neurological disease or condition is not an easy task. I believe WBV can help, but it needs to be used gently.

Overview of Neurological Diseases and WBV

There has been quite a lot of research on WBV and neurological conditions, using a wide variation in study protocols, but, in general, the studies gave elderly people with disease much more vibration than I, as an experienced natural health practitioner and practitioner of WBV, would give to that population. One study gave two vibration sessions per day, fifteen minutes per session, over a period of three days, to elderly people with Parkinson's (average age of seventy-four years), that's a total of seventy-five minutes of vibration in three days;[8] that is sixty times the dosage I feel is correct. I would start elderly people with Parkinson's at perhaps thirty seconds a few times a week at the lowest vibration setting on my gentlest machine. Even in younger people without such severe health issues, I generally see the best results starting with one minute and slowly building up over a period of several weeks to perhaps five minutes, depending on the individual.

In general, researchers are using too much vibration too soon, and they are using desynchronizing or otherwise stressful-for-the-mind vibration machines. For people with neurological diseases, lowering stress and optimizing the neurological effect is critical.

In addition, issues of detoxification and nutritional deficiencies and support should be addressed (see chapter 7), and I would recommend additional energy medicine, particularly homeopathy (see *Homeopathy Plus Whole Body Vibration: Combining Two Energy Medicines Ignites Healing*, by Becky Chambers).

To realize the potential benefits of WBV, especially in weakened populations of people who already have disease, the best results will be seen when you 1) start with slowly and gradually increasing duration and frequency of vibration, 2) use the proper type of vibration machine

The best results will be seen when you 1) start with slowly and gradually increasing duration and frequency of vibration, 2) use the proper type of vibration machine (low stress and synchronizing rather than desynchronizing), and 3) combine WBV with nutritional and energy medicine support.

(low stress and synchronizing rather than desynchronizing), and 3) combine it with nutritional and energy medicine support.

Brain Synchronization—A Missing Link?

Brain synchronization is the simultaneous, in-phase firing of brain cells across regions of the brain. These combined signals generate electromagnetic brain waves, which can be measured by electroencephalography (EEG) and magnetic resonance imaging (MRI).

How does this relate to WBV? Synchronized wavelengths from an outside source can cause "brain entrainment"—the synchronization of brain waves. This has been studied with sound and light and has been linked to increases in creativity, memory, learning, problem solving, and intuition, as well as to improvements in depression,

Certain types of whole body vibration deliver a synchronized message into the nervous system that may similarly lead to brain entrainment. As any engineer can attest, it is impossible to ever completely synchronize two motors; whereas one motor can produce a completely smooth and synchronized vibration (see pages 114–123). Some types of vibration machines can create a desynchronizing message that your nervous system will transmit to your brain with potentially negative consequences. This opposite state, asynchronous brain-wave activity, has been linked to disease states such as ADD, schizophrenia, depression, traumatic brain injury, and others.

anxiety, and ADHD.[vi] Biofeedback, for example, takes advantage of brain entrainment to treat mental and physical health issues. There are now numerous companies promoting sound entrainment CDs for better brain function.

Synchronized brain waves seem to foster the formation of new synaptic connections, or brain plasticity and learning. Earl Miller, the Picower Professor of Neuroscience at MIT and the senior author of a study published in *Neuron* in June 2014, has been studying the effects of brain synchronization. According to Dr. Miller in an interview with the MIT news office, he has found that "the phenomenon of brain-wave synchronization likely precedes the changes in synapses, or connections between neurons, believed to underlie learning and long-term memory formation."[9]

"The phenomenon of brain-wave synchronization likely precedes the changes in synapses, or connections between neurons, believed to underlie learning and long-term memory formation."

Brain plasticity (the formation of new connections between brain cells) has been known for some time now to be a critical element for learning. However, brain plasticity, meaning the actual growth of neurons, takes too long to account for the human mind's flexibility. How the brain can process and utilize new information almost instantly has remained a mystery. As Miller explains, "Plasticity doesn't happen on that

[vi]There have been many studies to back these claims. Please see the "Brain Synchronization" section under Additional Research Studies at the back of the book.

kind of time scale. The human mind can rapidly absorb and analyze new information as it flits from thought to thought. These quickly changing brain states may be encoded by synchronization of brain waves across different brain regions."[10]

Miller further describes the link between brain-wave resonance and brain development with an intriguing allusion to separate voices joining together; that is, waves of sounds: "There is some unknown mechanism that allows these resonance patterns to form, and these circuits start humming together. That humming may then foster subsequent long-term plasticity changes in the brain, so real anatomical circuits can form. But the first thing that happens is they start humming together."[11]

Brain synchronization also increases with meditation. Dr. Joe Dispenza, an internationally known lecturer, researcher, and author, has been studying and mapping the brain waves of meditators for decades. He describes the effects of brain synchronization, or coherence, thus: "What syncs in the brain begins to link in the brain. Once your brain gets coherent, you get coherent. When it gets orderly, you get orderly, when it works well, you work well."[12]

Dr. Dispenza describes the opposite state—that is, asynchronous brain-wave activity—as one that "causes our brain waves to fire in a very disordered, incoherent pattern (which in turn means our bodies can't work efficiently). . . . the electrochemical messages or signals they are sending to different parts of the brain and body are mixed and erratic, so the body cannot then operate in a balanced, optimal state."[13]

Is Whole Body Vibration Working Like Meditation?

In recent years, there has been a surge of interest in meditation as an aid in healing, as science and medicine have shown meditation's effectiveness in improving mental and physical health. Over three thousand studies on mindfulness meditation have shown that it can improve sleep, help you lose weight, lower stress levels, decrease loneliness in seniors, improve attention, manage chronic pain, reduce stress and depression, treat binge eating and other eating disorders, and contribute to greater cell longevity. An important aspect of mindfulness meditation is to focus your attention on your body and be in the present moment—things that WBV is very good at helping you do; almost automatically, you will begin to do so as the vibration floods through your body.

WBV has not been studied as an aid to meditation, but logically and intuitively this idea makes sense. WBV is such a powerful physical sensation throughout every part of your body that it almost forces you to pay attention to your body—if you are not distracting yourself by watching TV or some other activity. Focusing your thoughts on your body connects your mind to your body and brings the mind into the present moment, as opposed to worrying about the many things we all find to obsess and worry about, in a similar way to mindfulness meditation.

Perhaps WBV is helping our brains move to a meditative state, and this meditative state is a guiding force in WBV's healing effect.

Brain entrainment methods, such as sound CDs and other repetitive calming stimuli, are also commonly used to help people meditate. If WBV is a form of brain entrainment, synching our brain waves, then perhaps WBV is also slowing our brain waves down as is seen with meditation. Perhaps WBV is helping our brains move to a meditative state, and this meditative state is a guiding force in WBV's healing effect. Research in this area, including mapping brain waves states while using WBV, could be enlightening.

In my twenty years of experience using WBV, I have had many people report that they almost immediately feel more alive, awake, and rejuvenated in their minds. They report suddenly tackling a project that seemed too difficult before—like writing reports and papers (in my case—books!)—and having improvements in mood, focus, concentration, and even memory. I am excited by the possibilities and plan to pursue research in this area as soon as possible.

Electromagnetic Chi Energy

Another part of the puzzle may be how WBV interacts with our electromagnetic life force energy—our chi. Every time you are on a vibration plate, all your neurons are activated, shooting electromagnetic energy through your body and brain; this electromagnetic energy is fundamentally connected to our physical and mental states. The electromagnetic nature of our brains is recognized by modern allopathic medicine; electroencephalography (EEG) measures electronic brain waves, and magnetic resonance imaging (MRI) creates images of the brain by measuring its electromagnetic energy.

On an even deeper level, quantum physics describes the world of subatomic particles that makes up all matter and from which electromagnetic energy arises. Quantum physicist Ervin Lazlo explains that science is in the midst of a "shift from matter to energy as the primary reality. . . . There is no categorical divide between the physical world, the living world, and the world of mind and consciousness."[14] Norman Shealy, MD, PhD, describes this connection thus: "A quantum universe is a set of probabilities, susceptible to influence by many factors, including thought, will, and intention."[15]

Our chi energy is created by our thoughts and emotions—in effect, an accumulation of our experiences and our emotions and thoughts about these experiences.[16, 17] Dr. Dispenza elaborates on how this process works:

> When we think a thought, those networks of neurons that fire in our brain create electrical charges. When those thoughts also cause a chemical reaction that results in a feeling or an emotion, as well as when a familiar feeling or emotion is driving our thoughts, those feelings create magnetic charges. They merge with the thoughts that create the electric charges to produce a specific electromagnetic field equal to your state of being.[18]

Many cultures throughout time have recognized the existence of a life-force energy. The Chinese call it chi, Indians call it prana, and European traditions have called it variously life force, soul, spirit, vital energy, vital principle, elan, and more. This energy guides and powers one's body and life, and disturbances in this energy due to trauma of any sort can have a profound effect on your physical and mental state.

Thousands of years ago, the Chinese discovered and mapped "energy meridians" in the body. Each of these energy pathways is associated with different organs and bodily systems. The Chinese medical system of acupuncture is based on maintaining a healthy and balanced flow of energy between those different meridians.

Ayurvedic medicine (developed thousands of years ago in India and still in use today) describes chakras, spinning energy vortexes in our bodies, that are also associated with particular body systems and organs. In fact, some people can sense their own vibrational energy, and when these people stand on a vibrating plate, they report feeling energy shooting through their energy meridians— and their chakras unblocking and spinning faster.

There is, in fact, measurable electromagnetic energy emanating from all things. This is because all substances are made from molecules that are, in turn, made from even smaller vibrating particles that have positive or negative electrical charges. Thus, every substance has an electromagnetic charge that can be measured with sensitive scientific equipment. For example, Kirlian photography can detect and record the electromagnetic wavelengths around a person or object.[19]

Piezoelectricity

In addition to causing our neurons to fire, WBV stimulates electromagnetic energy through a physical property of crystals called piezoelectricity—the ability of crystals to turn mechanical vibration into electrical vibration. Our bodies are living liquid crystals in the sense that we are highly organized molecular structures, and as such we have the property of piezoelectricity.

Shealy describes our "bodies, souls, minds, and emotional realm" as "a living matrix" with the property of piezoelectricity.[20] "Waves of mechanical vibration moving through the living matrix produce electrical fields and vice versa. . . . Connective tissue is a liquid crystalline semiconductor. Piezoelectric signals from the cells can travel throughout the body in this medium."[21] The result is that "energetic treatment of one part of this living matrix always affects the whole."[22]

Your body turns the mechanical vibration into the electrical energy vibrations you need to heal, balance, and unblock your energy system.

Every time you are on a vibration plate, your neurons fire, shooting electromagnetic energy through your body and brain; then your body turns the mechanical vibration into the electrical energy vibrations you need to heal, balance, and unblock your energy system. Energy flows into and through your energy meridians and chakra energy centers, increasing their proper spinning and energy flow. Since these energy meridians and chakras are linked to different organs, body systems, emotions, and needs, improving the flow of energy helps heal the physical body and mind and improve life—all at the same time.

Energy Medicine and Pain Management

Different forms of "energy medicine," such as acupuncture, tai chi, and homeopathy are also known for their ability to decrease pain.[23-26] Acupuncture is one of the more familiar of these methods in the United States. Dr. Norm Shealy, one of the early gurus of alternative health and a groundbreaking innovator in energy medicine, reports marked improvement—using acupuncture only—in 70 percent of people with rheumatoid arthritis who failed to improve with conventional medicine; 75 percent of people with migraines; 80 percent of people with diabetic neuropathy; 70 percent of people with depression; and 70 percent of people with chronic low back pain.[27]

In China, where acupuncture originated, surgeries are sometimes performed with only the aid of acupuncture. This is hard to believe, but I can say from personal experience that acupuncture does have a remarkable ability to control pain. I am very pain sensitive, usually requiring extra Novocain for the slightest dental procedure, yet I once had a tooth pulled using only acupuncture (this was during a period when my chemical sensitivities were severe, and I could not tolerate any Western-medicine drugs). Gripping the dental chair in great fear, to my amazement I felt only a wrenching, pulling sensation—no pain.

WBV is like acupuncture in its ability to lower pain and to stimulate our electromagnetic system.

WBV is like acupuncture in its ability to lower pain and to stimulate our electromagnetic system. I have seen hundreds of people step on a whole body vibration plate and get off one to two minutes later with their pain gone. The placebo effect is unlikely, as many of these people had never heard of vibration or its benefits, and I usually don't have time to mention this before they step onto the plate at the crowded expos where this often happens. But if WBV works like energy medicine, things that seem impossible might turn out to be possible after all.

TESTIMONIALS

I am a fifty-seven-year-old tradesman. After a lifetime of hard physical work, I had come to expect arthritic pain as a normal part of my workday. My ankles, knees, hips, and lower back jabbed at me constantly, and my response had been to tough it out. It was a losing proposition, and it appeared that hip replacement was inevitable.

When a friend offered to let me try her vibration machine, the skeptic in me thought "yeah, right." That was weeks ago. This morning, I scampered down the stairs like a teenager. The remarkable thing is that I felt relief after the first five-minute session. Now, I simply stand on my WBV machine for five minutes each morning and head off to work with a happy song in my heart. The pain has gone. Imagine that.

—*Wayne Young, master electrician, age 57*

I came to Becky with hip and back pain that had been getting progressively worse for four to five months, with no relief from either physical therapy or a chiropractor. I could barely get out of my car when I arrived and limped up to Becky's door. She had me stand on the vibration machine for only a few minutes and stretch out my hip, and my pain was gone! I jumped into my car with no problem!! I was amazed! After two weeks I could feel some discomfort starting up again and gave her a call. She told me I could keep coming to her for "treatments," or I could buy a machine for myself and be pain free on my own!!

So I bought my vibration machine and never looked back!! It has been several years and at sixty-three years old, I have no stiffness or pain at all. I believe it also helped with my balance, as I can do the yoga stand on one foot now and don't have any tripping/stumbling episodes anymore.

Recently, I had to put my machine away for three weeks while I got some work done in my house. I started getting numbness in my hands and stiff knees when I was in bed. I had to get that machine out to get relief! It is so easy to use—I have now worked up to ten minutes of vibration at a high frequency three times a week. Keep up the good work Becky! I can't live without my machine!!

—L. Allen, age 63

My Experience with Brain Desynchronization

To achieve greater power, thus a greater workout effect, many WBV machines have two motors in them. However, as any engineer can attest, it is impossible to ever completely synchronize two motors. This lack of complete synchronization in the message sent through your body by double-motor machines will have a desynchronizing effect on your nervous system and energy field, which can have negative consequences over time. While people cannot detect the millisecond lack of synchronization on a conscious level while on a WBV machine, your nervous system and energy fields are extremely sensitive, and, on a deeper, unconscious level, they will be picking up this message.

Health effects from this desynchronization can be difficult to recognize and detect, especially with strong healthy people. Since

A lack of complete synchronization in the message sent through your body by double-motor machines will have a desynchronizing effect on your nervous system and energy field, which can have negative consequences over time.

the athletes typically using this type of machine have such strong overall health, this side effect may go unnoticed for years. By the time trouble begins to develop (and since it involves the nervous system and brain which controls your entire body, it can show up as any type of problem), these users have seen so many positive effects that they do not suspect they may be using the wrong sort of vibration machine. But with older and otherwise more sensitive or fragile people, this effect can be seen much more quickly and dramatically. I believe this may be part of the explanation for why some research on WBV with older people and those with health issues has not been as good as was hoped for and expected based on early research with animals and healthy young athletes.

For me, as the sensitive canary in the mine, problems quickly become clear. After my first year with one of these double-motor machines, during which I did see improvements and became stronger than I had been in many years, my health suddenly deteriorated. I experienced a sudden and mysterious downturn and had such severe muscle weakness that I could not make it up the stairs or even across the room (this after having improved from years of debilitating health issues to climbing Mt. Washington only two weeks earlier). My allergies, chemical sensitivities, multiple infections, digestive distress, and nervous-system problems also all returned. It seemed to be linked to the vibration, somehow, as I would get much worse after the slightest amount, but what exactly about the vibration was bothering me was difficult to determine.

Dr. DeOrio, an early expert in WBV[28] and my doctor at that time, theorized that it was a desynchronization effect from the double-motor machine that was causing my sudden downturn. After much trial and error and eventually switching to a single motor machine, it became clear that he was correct; only desynchronizing vibration was causing problems, not single-motor vertical vibration, which provides a fully synchronized signal to one's nervous system. I have now been exclusively using single-motor vertical vibration machines for fifteen years without a problem. The always perfectly synchronized message from these machines helps your brain and neurological system to synchronize their electromagnetic signals, while still providing all the other benefits of vibration.

Thus, because double-motor machines can cause brain desynchronization, and because brain-wave synchronization and optimization are such powerful effects, I only recommend relatively calm and gentle single-motor, vertical (also called linear) vibration. Whole body vibration has many wonderful benefits, but the issue of brain synchronization and optimal brain functioning is critical to long-term benefits and health.

CHAPTER 6

Rejuvenation
Sex, Beauty, and Mobility

Feeling the Pain . . .

Oh, my achin' joints!

Getting old is no picnic! Sex loses its appeal, beauty becomes an expensive full-time project, and mobility is a creaky, painful exercise of adjusting to limitations.

But perhaps the fountain of youth does exist—and it vibrates!

WBV has numerous global rejuvenation effects, such as raising human growth hormone and testosterone,[1] increasing circulation to all cells, detoxification, muscle and nerve stimulation, and energy balancing. These effects help your body repair its tissues and functions, and the effects can be especially dramatic with sexual libido and performance, skin tone and color, body shape, cellulite and fat deposits, and joint flexibility, pain, and strength.

The photo of me on the following page (and in color on page 173) was taken last year at age fifty-nine. I have never had any sort of surgical or medical cosmetic procedure, and I once weighed

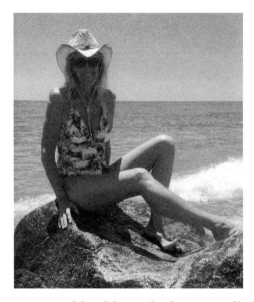

two hundred pounds, was severely and chronically depressed for thirty years, had an eating disorder, and had debilitating health problems in what seemed like every part of my body.

I am now happier, healthier, more creative and productive than I've ever been and have no significant health issues. All I can say is, natural health methods, especially whole body vibration, nutrition, and homeopathy (an energy medicine), have an incredible ability to help you change your life.

Consider the case of cats. Cats have "nine lives" . . . and they purr—essentially a built-in whole body vibration system. Cats purr, or vibrate, when they are happy but also when they are sick or stressed. Cats generally have strong bones and joint health throughout most of their lives, allowing them to survive falls that no other animal can;[vii] they have an amazing ability to heal injured bones, muscles, tendons, ligaments, and joints; and they can usually bounce back rapidly from other illnesses. Is purring the root of the myth that cats have nine lives . . . ?[2]

[vii]Researchers who looked at the records of 132 cat falls from an average height of five and a half stories found that 90 percent had survived. The record height for a cat falling and surviving is forty-five stories.

Testosterone

WBV has been shown to increase levels of the sex hormone testosterone.[3-7] Normally, as men get older, their testosterone levels gradually decline—typically by about 1 percent per year after age thirty. Meanwhile, women have testosterone levels of about 10 percent of men's to begin with, and their testosterone levels drop rapidly at menopause. Testosterone, the major sex hormone for males, is closely linked to libido and sexual performance, as well as overall energy levels. Testosterone is also important for women.

To understand about the function of testosterone in the female body, there is no greater expert than Susan Rako, MD, a psychiatrist, who wrote a groundbreaking book in 1996, *The Hormone of Desire: The Truth about Testosterone, Sexuality, and Menopause* (updated in 1999, still in print, and still the most comprehensive and accurate body of information about the physiology and function of testosterone in women's bodies). In it, she describes her experience, and the research, that has shown that testosterone levels affect libido (meaning one's "life force," not just sexual drive) for both

WBV has been shown to increase levels of the sex hormone testosterone. . . . Testosterone, the major sex hormone for males, is closely linked to libido and sexual performance, [and it] is also important for women.

men and women. In Dr. Rako's words, testosterone is "essential . . . to the healthy functioning of virtually all tissues in [a woman's] body and to her experience of vital energy and sexual libido."[8] Typical high-testosterone effects include focused motivation, assertiveness, a sense of power, and enhanced sex drive. Healthy levels of testosterone help women take risks and live their lives with exuberance.

Testosterone also has powerful anti-aging effects. It turns fat into muscle, keeps skin supple, increases bone-mineral density, gives us a positive mood, and boosts our ability to handle stress. It supports mental health and cognitive functioning, also liver function and blood-vessel health. Low testosterone levels have been associated with heart attack, Alzheimer's disease, osteoporosis, and depression.

> **Testosterone is "essential . . . to the healthy functioning of virtually all tissues in [a woman's] body and to her experience of vital energy and sexual libido."**

There are drugs, such as Androgel, designed to raise testosterone in men, but as is generally true with prescription drugs, there are side effects[9] (and women and children must carefully avoid contact with these gels, or their hormone balances may be thrown off). The list of common side effects for men include nausea, vomiting, headache, dizziness, hair loss, trouble sleeping, change in sexual desire, redness/swelling of the skin, change in skin color, or acne.

Unlikely but serious side effects can also occur—breast pain/enlargement, swelling of the feet/ankles, weight gain, very slow/shallow/difficult breathing, and/or weakness. And rare but very serious side effects include trouble urinating, mental/mood changes (e.g., depression, agitation, hostility), change in size/shape of the testicles, testicular pain/tenderness, stomach/abdominal pain, dark urine, change in the amount of urine, yellowing of eyes/skin, calf tenderness/swelling/pain. Why risk all this when there is a safe, natural approach that has many *positive* "side effects"?

While testosterone in the form of gels, creams, or pills is sometimes prescribed for women, the long-term safety of testosterone drug therapy for women is unknown. At this time, no commonly prescribed testosterone preparations have been approved by the Food and Drug Administration for use in women. If a testosterone drug is prescribed for women, it is off label and not tested for safety.

WBV will not raise testosterone levels too high or too fast or interact negatively with other drugs or bodily functions. WBV promotes the body's ability to achieve its highest natural state of health. This is not to say that WBV is totally without risk. There are contraindications (see chapter 8), and it is important to understand detoxification and nutrition, but as a natural therapy, WBV promotes the optimal natural functioning of all body organs and systems.

Human Growth Hormone

Another important benefit of WBV is increased levels of human growth hormone (HGH), which promote the healing of tissues critical for joint health and mobility (ligaments, tendons, muscles, bones, and nerves) along with all other tissues. HGH levels typically fall with age, and any method of

Another important benefit of WBV is increased levels of HGH, which promote the healing and rejuvenation of all tissues.

raising them is hotly pursued by those interested in rejuvenation of any sort, whether it is for athletic performance, daily pain relief and function, sexual libido and function, or beauty.

Early research (2000) showed promising results with WBV, giving an increase in HGH levels of up to 150 percent.[10–13] Several recent studies have since then confirmed increases of HGH with WBV.[14–16]

Other WBV Effects That Improve Libido and Sex

WBV also raises serotonin (see chapter 5), a neurotransmitter in the brain that is important for mood and the ability to experience pleasure, including sexual pleasure. Plus, confidence and a good mood go a long way toward improving sexual experiences. The increase in strength and physical energy levels associated with WBV will also help with sexual performance.

Another critical area affecting sexuality is your chi energy. Every time you are on a vibration plate, because of the piezoelectrical ability of the human body that converts mechanical vibration into electromagnetic energy (as described in chapter 5), you will be sending energy through the entire chakra system, and all of that energy will pass through the Kundalini chakra—the seat of your most basic survival needs, including sexual energy.

People who are sensitive to this energy can sometimes actually feel their chakras spinning. When these clients or people I meet at expos stand on a vibrating plate, their eyes glaze over with delight, and they talk about feeling energy shooting through meridians, and chakras unblocking and spinning faster.

Whether people can identify "energy" or not, I've observed humorous situations develop when people try a vibration machine at expos. Some people end up suddenly feeling *very good indeed*, and the more uninhibited ones are not shy about expressing themselves with sexy ohhs and ahhhs—leading strangers up and down the aisles to turn to see what all the laughing is about. Since this happens even with very gentle vibration where you cannot physically feel the vibration past your knees, and it happens quickly (in thirty to sixty seconds), it seems that at least some of this reaction is due to electromagnetic energy transmitting through the body, rather than hormonal or direct physical stimulation.

My favorite story of increasing libido and sexual enjoyment involves a sixty-year-old woman who came to me twice a week for three weeks. She was primarily interested in losing weight and increasing bone density. Her husband, though, was quite skeptical, "So, you think you are going to lose weight and increase bone density just by standing on that machine?!" After three weeks, my client came to me and said, "I think those hormonal affects you were talking about might be kicking in. . . . Now my husband says, '*Buy one.*'"

Beauty

Beauty is mostly health and happiness radiating through our bodies. Since WBV is fantastic for your physical and emotional health, you will be beautiful, too. Working out with vibration will tone your body, balance hormones, increase neurotransmitters in your brain, help you lose fat and cellulite, increase circulation to all tissues (resulting in increased collagen production which tightens and smooths skin), and put color in your cheeks and a sparkle in your eyes. When you feel good, you take better care of yourself: eating wisely, exercising more, maybe even sprucing up your wardrobe and changing your hairstyle. Then you get more recognition for your contributions, because now you're more effective and radiating confidence, and you feel even better! It's like a snowball rolling downhill—it just keeps getting bigger all the time.

While cellulite and wrinkles are normal signs of aging, with improved health, they can be delayed and/or decreased. Cellulite is the lumpy appearance of fat that develops primarily in women, much to their annoyance, especially on the thighs, knees, backside, and upper arms. But cellulite is not really a fat problem, and it has nothing to do with how much you weigh. Cellulite is made up of a special type of fat, called "subcutaneous," that is within the skin layer, and it can't be burned as fuel, so you don't lose it by dieting.

As we age, circulation begins to decrease (especially to the thighs and other cellulite-prone areas) due to blood-vessel damage and the effects of decreasing estrogen. Poor circulation leads to a lack of nutrients and more toxins building up in the skin, which further damages blood vessels and lowers collagen production (the major component of a connective-tissue support structure that holds the subcutaneous fat in place). All this means that fat bulges out through the spaces between the fibers of that collagen-support structure, creating the lumpy effect. In other words, as one doctor put it, your backside is something like an old mattress with the stuffing bulging out!

Wrinkles are due to the loss of subcutaneous fat that, together with a healthy connective-tissue structure, usually plumps out and smooths skin. This, along with the loss of elastin—which gives skin its flexibility, allowing it to stretch and give without damage—results in wrinkles.

WBV increases circulation, thus attacking the root cause of cellulite and wrinkles. Increased circulation brings more nutrients to the skin, causing greater collagen production, which strengthens the connective-tissue structure holding that unruly subcutaneous fat in place. Meanwhile, those nasty toxins and their associated free-radical damage are flushed out, further helping your skin to glow and retain its youthful appearance. WBV also increases human growth hormone,[17–20] which promotes the healing of all tissues, including connective tissue and skin cells. Hop on a vibration machine, and you are fighting the "do not go gently into that good night" battle on all fronts.

WBV increases circulation, thus attacking the root cause of cellulite and wrinkles.

Add in good nutrition and nutritional supplements, and you have fresh troops pouring over the hills laden with supplies to fight that battle. Protein sources contain keratin, a building block for collagen and elastin, and antioxidants (from fruits and vegetables) neutralize free-radical damage from toxins. Anti-aging creams are available now with these very ingredients incorporated into them, but keep in mind that nutrients are much more effectively absorbed into cells from the bloodstream than through the skin.

Also, be sure to get plenty of potassium—ideally from fruit, which also has very low sodium. This maintains the proper electrolyte balance, which promotes good hydration of your cells. Don't forget to also consume lots of omega 3 oils, as they have many beneficial anti-aging effects, including strengthening cell-wall integrity. This internal balancing and tweaking of our hydration system is a more effective approach than hydrating the skin with lotions. Of course, you can always do both, lotions and nutrition; just don't forget the healthy food. As your mother said, "Eat your vegetables!"

Mobility

One of the most well-known and accepted uses of WBV is for physical therapy, and WBV is used in physical therapy centers around the world. Sports franchises and top athletes use WBV for athletic training and to help the athletes heal faster from injuries. They are also less likely to be injured in the first place because their joints are stronger.

WBV is effective therapy for a wide range of joint and movement issues, including arthritis, bursitis, tendonitis, fibromyalgia, pulled and strained muscles, weakness, range-of-motion issues, and poor flexibility.

WBV is effective therapy for a wide range of joint and movement issues.

One of the most obvious physical therapy benefits of WBV is that working out on a WBV plate is strength training without lifting weights or stressing the joints, since you don't have to move on the vibration plate to work muscles. By holding different positions on the plate, you can target different muscles and joints (see pages 151–172 for illustrations), and the intensity of the workout and stress on the joints can be adapted to varying levels of mobility, strength, and function.

Flexibility also increases, especially when stretching positions are used, due to the automatic reflex response causing rapid involuntary tightening and relaxing of muscles. Muscle fibers will automatically tense and relax at the same rate as the vibration, twenty to fifty times per second, and the relaxation phase of this response rapidly and gently increases flexibility.

The automatic reflex response has a massaging effect as well as a stretching effect that, along with relaxing tight muscles, increases circulation, bringing nutrients to the affected areas to aid in repair and regrowth. This massage effect happens automatically, but it can be heightened by placing the affected part of the body on the plate and relaxing. For example, one of my favorite positions, for pure enjoyment and relaxation, is a calf massage, where you lie down on your back, place your calves on the plate, cross your hands behind your head, and zone out. To get the full massage effect it is important to just rest that body part on the plate—to not be holding weight, as that will cause the muscles automatically to work to hold that weight up. So standing on the plate is quite different from laying different parts of your body on the plate.

These stretching and massage effects can have rapid results. I have seen many people get on a machine and find that by the time they get off a few minutes later, painfully tight muscles have loosened, and they have a greater range of motion.

Balance also improves, because specialized nerve clusters that control balance (called proprioceptors) are stimulated, along with the rest of the nervous system. This is of particular benefit to the elderly, who are at risk of dangerous falls.

Scientific Research

A recent and very large systematic review of WBV and human gait analyzed forty-six clinical trials involving a total of 2,029 patients.[21] Looking at several measures of gait—such as the "Timed Up-and-Go" (TUG) test, the "six-minute walking test" (6MWT), and the "ten-meter walking test" (10MWT), among others—they analyzed the combined data from studies mostly with postmenopausal women and the elderly. Also included were studies on people who had strokes, MS, other neurological conditions, knee osteoarthritis, and/or chronic obstructive pulmonary disease (COPD), and children with a several different pathologies.

After analyzing all the data, they concluded that WBV had some positive results, especially for otherwise healthy elderly people. For this population, there was a "strong level of evidence that WBV can improve mobility by improving the TUG test, and gait speed by improving the 10MWT."[22] Translated, this means that WBV training can help balance and gait speed in the elderly.[23] This did not include "gait quality" for the elderly—so you will get there quicker, though you still may not be graceful.

In this survey, they also found improved walking performance for stroke sufferers and in patients with knee osteoarthrosis, but not for balance in stroke and multiple sclerosis patients. Most of the studies with children resulted in improved measures of gait.

They did not draw positive conclusions for the other conditions, determining that there was either no improvement or too much variability; but I feel that with the proper machines and dosages, it might be possible to improve these outcomes also.

Vibrant Health's 2019 WBV Survey

In our survey, we asked respondents (a total of fifty-three, 88 percent of whom were fifty to eighty years of age) to rate their mobility before and after they had begun to use WBV, on a scale of 1 to 5 (1 = poor, 5 = excellent). Using Vibrant Health machines, survey subjects reported an average 20 to 28 percent improvement in mobility, strength, and energy levels, along with an average 31 percent decrease in pain, within a few months of beginning their WBV program. Improvements often began within a few days. We did not ask respondents whether they had any diagnosed neurological conditions, so we cannot say our data shows improvement with neurological diseases, but our data does show improved mobility with older people.

Using Vibrant Health machines, survey subjects reported an average 20–28 percent improvement in mobility, strength, and energy levels, along with an average 31 percent decrease in pain. Improvements often began within a few days.

Our survey is a testimony to my method. It is not meant to be a clinical trial but rather to be a guide for future research.

Pain and Inflammation

Pain and inflammation often drop rapidly using WBV, sometimes after just one session of one or two minutes (see chapter 4). When used properly, there can be almost instant reductions in pain and inflammation; this may be due to WBV's effects on the electromagnetic system, as they happen too fast to attribute to other causes.

Pain and inflammation levels often drop rapidly using WBV, sometimes after just one session of one or two minutes.

Significant relief within days may reflect changes in our brain waves, increasing our brain's ability to guide our body toward healing.

To achieve lasting pain reduction, however, most people will require regular sessions (usually two to three times per week) for at least a couple of months. But, like exercise and for lifelong health, the ideal way to use WBV is to incorporate it into your life as a part of your daily routine. This is easy, since it is quick, feels great, and supplies instant gratification as well as long-term benefits.

TESTIMONIALS

Sometimes mobility problems are due to nerve issues, such as with diabetic neuropathy or other conditions. Because WBV is calming, anti-inflammatory, and stimulates the regeneration of the nervous system (see chapter 5), there can be dramatic results. One of my clients, Richard Hawkins, a retired orthopedic surgeon, had been a lifelong runner before he lost his ability to run due to a mysterious nerve issue. He had been in pain and unable to run for seven years when he met me.

I suspected mercury poisoning, as he had been eating tuna fish every day for thirty years, and mercury is a potent neurotoxin. I suggested some heavy metal detox products, a few homeopathics, diet changes, and vibration. From the very first session of vibration (one minute), he noticed an improvement, and within a few weeks of twice-a-week, short sessions, he had begun to jog to his car with a big grin.

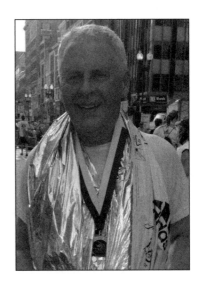

A lifelong runner, I gave up running at age sixty after developing numbness and pain in both feet. I spent seven years unable to run at all. I went to many different doctors, including specialists who told me there was nerve damage, and I would never get better, and I even tried surgery—all with no improvement.

Then four years ago, I met Becky and started vibrating, increasing eventually to twenty minutes daily. I saw an improvement after the first session, and there has been a steady increase in function and feeling ever since. Now, four years later, I have just successfully completed this year's Boston Marathon, my twenty-seventh, at the age of seventy. Thanks, Becky!

—Richard Hawkins, retired orthopedic surgeon, age 71

I am in my seventies and a regular tennis player, but I have a shoulder injury from a bicycle accident years ago that never fully healed, and it has bothered me ever since. After only two weeks of vibration twice a week, it is getting a lot better. I would say it is 90 percent improved.

—*Robert Williams, retired engineer, age 74*

I'm seventy years old, and I've had increasing pain and stiffness in my legs for the last seven years. I started using Becky's vibration machine, and every time I use it for just a few minutes, my mind and body feel rejuvenated, and the pain in my legs goes away. And if I use the vibration after my regular exercise, the post exercise pain I usually have goes away. I feel like I am getting my younger body and self back.

—*Gene M., age 70*

I have had a severe case of restless leg syndrome for the past five to six years. During a twelve-week study at an area sleep clinic, my legs moved approximately 490 times per hour. Although I have tried several medications, all made me tired during my waking hours and were not very effective.

Since using your vibrating device, I find that I am sleeping more soundly and have discontinued taking my script for Provigil (a medication for shift workers and airline pilots), which helped me to focus and remain alert during the day. I have now been using WBV for over ten years, and it has continued to alleviate my restless leg syndrome and help me relax so that I can sleep. Thank you for introducing this new technology to Cynthia and me.

—*Brian Cichella, age 77*

CHAPTER 7

Detoxing and Lymphatic Drainage

The lymphatic system is a network of vessels, nodes, and organs that fights infections and removes waste products and toxins from our bodies. This system relies on passive circulation. In other words, unlike the blood vessels (which require a heart to pump the blood around the body), there is no pump for the lymph system. The lymph system relies on your muscles tightening and relaxing around the lymph vessels to move the lymph, a process called lymph drainage. To keep this system working well, it is important to be using your muscles regularly—another benefit of WBV!

Our immune system is our defense against infections of all sorts, so keeping your tissues well supplied with lymph is critical to your health and well-being. Inflammation levels, which are mediated in part by your immune system, can decrease with WBV (see chapter 4). This is indirect evidence that WBV is affecting your immune system. There have also been some studies directly showing an increase in immune-system infection-fighting cells with WBV.[1, 2]

Many people think they should use powerful high amplitude vibration to get as much of a lymphatic drainage effect as possible. *Do not do that.* Slow and steady is the best approach. Too much detoxing too quickly will make you worse. This problem is more common than many realize, especially when using vibration machines with people who already have health problems.

Liberating toxins from where they are relatively safely stored in your body causes a sudden increase in work for your detox organs (liver and kidneys primarily), putting a strain on already overworked and stressed organs. This can lead to increased symptoms instead of relief. I have seen "detoxing overload" situations innumerable times, and have experienced it myself.

You do not need high amplitude vibration for lymphatic drainage and detoxing—any vibration that travels throughout your entire body will be effective for this. In twenty years of using vibration, I have *never* had a person *not* get enough detoxification, including clients with lymphedema (a sometime painful swelling of arms or legs as lymph builds up in the tissues) and lipedema (causing an accumulation of excess fat in the legs)—two conditions for which improving lymphatic drainage is particularly important.

The position you hold on the plate determines which muscles are activated, so I advise using a variety of positions. Standing on the plate will activate the muscles in your lower body and torso but not your arms if you are standing upright. To increases lymphatic drainage in your arms, do some exercise positions where your hands are on the plate, such as push-ups.

With a very gentle vibration, where you cannot feel the vibration in your upper body, it would be advisable to also sit on the plate and place your hands on the plate, leaning your body weight on your arms to get more vibration into your upper body.

Toxins Everywhere

Our environment is loaded with toxins, and despite our best attempts to avoid them, some of these toxins will end up in our bodies. In a PBS television special several years ago, Bill Moyers, as a typical healthy person, had his blood tested at Mt. Sinai School of Medicine. Eighty-four different and highly toxic chemicals were found in his body.[3]

Once in our bodies, toxins may cause damage and disease. Toxins have been linked to almost all chronic health issues. Sherry A. Rogers, MD, a leading authority on environmental medicine, writes in her 2002 book, *Detoxify or Die:*

> Pesticides, volatile organic hydrocarbons, auto and industrial pollution, mycotoxins, heavy metals, and more mimic any disease. They can cause any symptom or disease from high blood pressure, heart failure, osteoporosis, high cholesterol, arthritis, or Alzheimer's disease to fibromyalgia, degenerating disks, Parkinson's disease, depression, fatigue, irritable bowel, loss of libido, colitis, asthma, eczema, prostatitis, esophagitis, atrial fibrillation, GERD (gastroesophageal reflux disease), hearing loss, headaches, recurrent sinus, ear or throat infections, diabetes or cancer, and more.[4]

What Should One Do?

A regular detoxification program is a wise idea for everybody, and it is essential for people with chronic health issues. Remember, however, that detoxification should be done with caution, as detoxing is stressful for the body and can cause an increase in symptoms for someone with an already weakened body. Your body has natural systems to eliminate and neutralize toxins through the colon, liver, kidneys, lymphatic system, lungs, and skin. However, with the buildup of toxicity levels in your body and the consequent breakdown of health, it is important to support and aid your body in this process.

A key benefit of vibration is that it is a powerful aid to your natural detoxification process. When vibrating, all your muscle fibers will involuntarily tense and relax at the same rate the machine is vibrating, twenty to fifty times per second. This process creates a powerful massage for your lymphatic system, which is one of the body's primary natural detoxing tools. Unlike the heart and blood, the lymph system does not have its own pumping system; muscles contracting around lymphatic vessels force the lymph (a clear fluid) to move. Thus the muscle workout provided by WBV leads to an increased flow of the lymph moving toxins out of your body. In addition, increased circulation brings more nutrients and oxygen to all the cells, helping them to function at a higher

The muscle workout provided by WBV leads to an increased flow of the lymph moving toxins out of your body; [also the] increased circulation brings more nutrients and oxygen to all the cells.

level and therefore dump more toxins and waste products into the lymphatic system.

Detox Overload

Detoxing with WBV is so powerful that it is an important limiting factor for many people using WBV—not muscle strength as many people assume. Detoxing will happen anytime you are on a machine, whether you just stand there or are actively exercising. As with detoxing after a massage or sauna or any other detox system, it is possible to overload your already-stressed detox pathways and have a temporary increase in symptoms. Common detox symptoms are exhaustion, headaches, and digestive problems, but any health issue that is linked to toxins can temporarily worsen as more toxins are released into the circulatory system. In fact, as any health problem you already have is a "weak link" in your system, when you stress your body with too much detoxing, that weak link is a likely place to show the strain.

Detox problems often do not show up until six to twenty-four hours after using WBV. So . . . use caution!

Candida yeast problems are also likely to flare up with detox overload. Since the liver is your major detox organ and is part of the immune system, under the increased strain, your immune system may temporarily weaken, and this opportunistic parasite may increase. In fact, a *Candida* yeast flare-up is a sign that you are in detox overload and need to do less vibration and possibly take a detox support supplement. Detox reactions are an enlightening opportunity to see the close connection between toxins and chronic health issues, something that is not always recognized by Western medicine.

Detox problems often do not show up until six to twenty-four hours after using WBV. So even though the vibration feels gentle and pleasant, use caution. Start slowly and increase slowly; many people will do best starting with just one minute the first day on a gentle, low-power machine (see chapter 9 for details on getting started).

What to Do If You Experience Detox Overload

If any existing symptoms worsen, or new ones suddenly appear, it is possible that toxins are involved. You should stop vibrating, rest a few days, and, if symptoms decrease, you can start up again with less vibration. You can aid your body with detoxing by drinking extra water and/or juice to help flush out toxins and by getting plenty of sleep. Additionally, you can try any of the following:

- ◆ Activated charcoal: Take two to six capsules two to three times per day. Be sure to take this product on an empty stomach (one hour before food or two hours after food), because it will absorb nutrients as well as toxins.

- ◆ Modified citrus pectin: This comes in powder or capsule form, so take one scoop (or six capsules) once a day. This is a great product (sold under several different brand names; I usually use PectaSol) that will be absorbed into your bloodstream, go everywhere in your body, and absorb only toxins. It can be taken with or without food.

- ◆ Protoclear: This is an excellent liver-supporting nutritional powder that combines many detox support nutrients, herbs, and PectaSol. Take one scoop once a day.

Consult with a natural healthcare practitioner for your specific situation. Sometimes additional products and/or homeopathic remedies are needed to resolve a situation.

CHAPTER 8

Choosing a Whole Body Vibration Machine

Over the last twenty years, I have used and sold a lot of different vibration machines. I have seen, with myself and from working with hundreds of clients, that the type of machine you use, especially with seniors (and others with health challenges), is critical to the success of whole body vibration. Since problems can develop from using the wrong machine (see below), I am careful which whole body vibration machines I use and recommend. Several years ago, using my knowledge and experience, I decided to develop my own machines to ensure that I always have available the best type of machines. Check my website (www.BCVibrantHealth.com) for the latest information.

Double-Motor Vibration Machine

As discussed earlier, to achieve greater power and thus a greater workout effect, many whole body vibration (WBV) machines have two motors in them. Seniors, especially, require a different approach than a "football player" mentality. Just as you wouldn't start a football training program at age sixty, or if you were young but had a neurological or skeletal muscular problem, you shouldn't use these double motor machines, either.

Additionally, because two motors can send a desynchronizing message into the nervous system, which can cause brain desynchronization (see page 85), I do not recommend this type of machine for anyone. Devastating effects can result. In my case, I suddenly developed extreme muscle weakness, bone pain, multiple infections, and a return of my allergies, chemical sensitivities, digestive and nervous-system problems, among other issues. It took me years to recover. The greater workout is not worth the risk. *Do not use a dual-motor machine!*

Interestingly, the proper type of vibration machine—vibration that sent a gentle and fully synchronized signal into my brain—aided me in my recovery. With this type of machine, I eventually fully recovered. I have been using this type of vibration for fifteen years now, and I only get better—mentally and physically!

Different Models and Makes

There are many companies now selling vibration machines, with some machines sold by many different distributors under different names, sometimes for widely varying prices; it can be hard to know exactly what type of vibration you are buying. There are also different terms used for important features of vibration machines, and sometimes the same word is used to refer to opposite things. I will try to clarify the situation.

Vibration machines were first developed (and are still best known) for their ability to create an intense workout. Many WBV-machine companies have the football mindset that the more power the better. Thus, many of the best-selling machines, and most of the machines you will find in health clubs and sports centers, are of the double-motor variety. Beyond this issue, there are several other variables to consider: direction of movement, frequencies, amplitudes, power (g-force), durability, and cost. Read further for a more complete discussion of these factors.

The most important information for many people is that you don't need to spend a great deal of money to get enormous benefit. There is a huge range of machines, and you can get an effective and therapeutic device for less than a gym membership and much less than what you might spend on healthcare. Considering all the benefits to your health, you will likely end up saving a great deal of money.

Direction of Movement

There are two major types of motion for vibration plates. Vertical, or linear, motion machines vibrate mostly up and down. This is the type of machine that I recommend for most people. As long as the vibration is produced with only one motor, this will provide a completely synchronized movement and message to your system, and this motion is the most stabilizing for your structural system.

Confusingly, variations of this first basic type of motion are produced by different motor configurations. The different motor

Vertical, or linear, motion machines vibrate mostly up and down.

types confer small amounts of horizontal motion and circular movement to the plate, along with a predominantly vertical motion. To seem different (and better), companies come up with different names, such as three-dimensional, horizontal, spiral, circular, triplanar, triangular, tri-phasic, multidimensional, omniflex, and piston. All these terms are describing basically the same type of motion.

There is, however, a great variation in amplitudes, g-force, durability, and cost with these machines. (There are usually a range of frequency [speed] settings on any given vertical vibration machine, but these frequency ranges are generally similar between machines of this type. See page 119 for more details on the relationship between the amplitude, frequency, and g-force [power] of the vibration.)

The intensity of your vibration workout depends on the power, or gravitational force (g-force), of the vibration—a factor that takes into account the amplitude and frequency of the machine, and weight (your own weight) that your muscles must hold against the vibration. As amplitudes, frequency, and your weight all can vary greatly, there is great flexibility in the intensity of your workout. To get a sense of what I mean by g-force, imagine putting your hand on a purring cat versus holding a jackhammer—these are very different experiences because of the different amplitudes and weights. A jackhammer's amplitude of vibration, and its weight, are much greater than those of a hand resting on a purring cat, so even though the frequencies of these vibrations are similar, the total g-force, and therefore effect, is greater for the jackhammer.

A second major type of vibration machine utilizes oscillation across a fulcrum in the middle of the plate, so that the plate rises

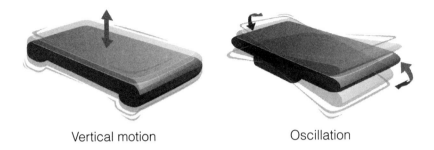

Vertical motion   Oscillation

and falls on either side like a child's seesaw. This motion is called oscillation, pivotal, or teeter-totter (in scientific research papers, this motion is also sometimes called sinusoidal[viii]). These machines usually have greater maximum amplitudes but lower frequencies. They can provide a good workout and high g-forces for less cost.

But the wild motion caused by essentially having a foot on each end of a rapidly moving seesaw can be destabilizing for your musculoskeletal system and stressful for your brain.

For ease of use and total health, I recommend a single-motor vertical-vibration machine with its perfect synchronization and smooth motion. While I believe that people of any age

A second major type of vibration machine utilizes oscillation across a fulcrum in the middle of the plate, so that the plate rises and falls on either side like a child's seesaw.

[viii]Even more confusingly, sinusoidal and "sinusoidal oscillation" is also sometimes used in scientific papers to mean any and all types of vibration, except "random" vibration. Sinusoidal describes an "S" curve, and if you graph the amplitude and frequency of vibration, unless it is a random frequency vibration, it will describe an S curve. So it can be, and often is in scientific papers, applied to all types of vibration, vertical and oscillating. The exception is "random" vibration with randomly changing frequencies, which is very seldom studied as a form of WBV. Another term sometimes used in research papers to refer to all non-random vibration is stochastic vibration.

should avoid machines that create stress and/or destabilization, I feel it is extra important for the elderly and anyone whose health, including brain health, is more vulnerable.

> **For ease of use and total health, I recommend a single-motor vertical-vibration machine with its perfect synchronization and smooth motion.**

There are now machines that have both types of motion available in one machine, and each is independently controlled. These machines are described as "dual motion" or "hybrid."

Don't confuse dual *motion* with dual *motor*. Dual motor refers to two motors operating at the same time, and, as I have stated, I recommend you always avoid this type of vibration (see above).

Dual motion machines have two motors and two motions, often with the option of operating both—at the same time. *Don't do that!* As long as only one motor is operating at a time, this is a viable option, though more expensive and not necessary. Oscillation vibration is not more effective in the long run for total health, and it is not as coherent and smooth a signal for the nervous system as single-motor vertical vibration.

The final type of machine is one in which a linear vibration motion is generated by sonic (sound) waves. No actual sound is produced by these machines; the term "sonic" is used here to describe a sound wave–type of mechanism that produces a vertical movement, not a sound. These machines typically can create smooth and synchronized vibrations with a range of amplitudes as well as frequencies, but the cost is also very high ($3,000–$10,000) without adding significant benefits.

Remember, more power does not mean better! Especially for seniors, the machines I most often recommend are $500 to $1,000.

Intense exercise is only one of many benefits you can get from vibration. For many people, if they try to work out too intensely with vibration at the beginning, they will end up feeling worse instead of better because of too much stress and detoxing. Be patient! Remember that you can get exercise many ways. The workout effect is not the only benefit, and it is not what makes vibration so unique. Muscle strength, toning, and weight loss are only the tip of the iceberg when it comes to vibration's benefits.

Remember, more power does not mean better! Especially for seniors, the machines I most often recommend are $500 to $1,000.

Gravitational (g) Force, Amplitude, and Frequency

The power of a machine (g-force) is determined by the amplitude (the distance the plate moves), the frequency (the rate or speed of vibration), and the weight of the person on the plate.[ix] The greater the amplitude, the frequency, and the weight, the greater the g-force. Again, imagine putting your hand on a purring cat versus holding a jackhammer—these are very different experiences because of the different amplitudes and weights involved, even

---

[ix]G-force is measured and expressed in g units that, for simplicity, will be implied but not written out in this book. For example, 0.3 g maximum g-force becomes 0.3 maximum g-force.

though the frequencies of vibration are similar. G-force is a popular and handy way to compare machines, though it is not an exact method, as the weight of different people varies significantly, and this is also a factor in determining g-force.

Changing the amplitude dramatically changes the g-force; with a low amplitude vibration feeling like the purring cat versus high amplitude machines that can rattle your body with their more jack-hammer-type vibration. To change the amplitude, one usually needs to change machines.

G-force and amplitude have become a hot topic, with many consumers searching for high numbers. This market pressure has led to some companies artificially inflating g-force and amplitude numbers. It is like women's dress sizes—we get bigger, but dress sizes stay the same or go down . . . because that is what we want!

In response to people wanting high-amplitude (high-power) machines and making buying decisions based on this factor, some companies use a peak-to-peak measurement of amplitude versus the standard centerline-to-peak amplitude measurement. Using the peak-to-peak-measurement method produces amplitudes twice as big as the centerline method, without actually changing the true vibration. Other companies deal with this issue by not posting amplitude information online at all. When amplitude information is posted online, there is no explanation as to which measurement is being referenced.

Double-motor, linear-motion machines can deliver high amplitudes, frequencies, and g-forces, but (as I noted earlier) I don't recommend these machines, and they are expensive, ranging from

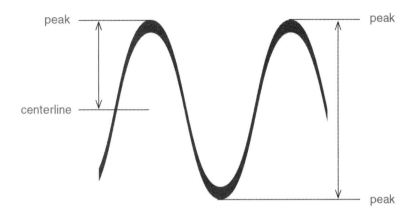

$3,500–$10,000. Oscillating motion machines have even higher amplitudes, but since the motion is so wild, the frequency is much lower. The resulting maximum g-forces can go quite high with these machines, but not as high as the maximum g-forces in double-motor vertical-vibration machines.

Most machines have a wide range of frequency (speed) settings. Linear vibration machines have settings ranging around 20–50 Hz (vibrations per second). Oscillation machines typically have lower frequency ranges (often 1–20 Hz).

Much effort has gone into figuring out which frequencies and types of motion are the best for losing weight and cellulite, increasing bone density and muscle strength, lymph drainage, etc. My experience is that focusing on exactly what frequency is the best for achieving certain effects is usually a moot point. By far the most important issue is to start at a low frequency and increase slowly so that you lower inflammation and stress, allowing your body and mind to heal itself.

However, as you become able to tolerate the higher frequencies, they are beneficial, and they do have more powerful effects. *Always go slowly,* or you may end up disappointed and stop entirely! Remember that even gentle vibration will be affecting your whole body, so no matter what frequency you use, you will be on your way to achieving the desired results. See chapter 9 for specific recommendations on getting started and for specific health issues.

Durability

This depends on the quality of construction. Plastic parts are not as durable as steel, but for low-cost, low–g-force machines, plastic can be a reasonable option. Larger, more powerful machines are usually made of steel and can weigh quite a lot. Many machines are made overseas and shipped to the US. Quality can vary widely, so be sure to check the warranty terms and weight limits for users. Generally, the higher the g-force and amplitude of a machine, the larger, heavier, and more expensive it is likely to be. This is because the motor must be more powerful to generate the greater amplitude, and since vibration tends to shake things apart, the machine must be built to withstand increasing force.

Cost

There is an enormous range in the cost of machines. You can spend anywhere from $200 for an inexpensive, cheaply made oscillation or vertical vibration machine, to $13,000 for some vibration machines, and everything in between. The cost depends on many factors, including the type of machine and amount of power, the quality of construction, availability of knowledgeable customer support services, demand, and the marketing strategy—the same machine made in Asia is selling in different places for a tenfold difference in price. Note, when checking out different machines, how exactly the same some "different" plates look. On the other hand, there are also copycat machines for sale; inferior, cheaply made machines that have been carefully designed to look very similar to expensive ones—it is like the Wild West out there.

For seniors, I recommend several different companies making and selling machines (see below). These are all excellent machines, very effective and therapeutic, delivering very smooth, synchronized, vertical vibration. In the comparisons below, I will outline the features of these machines, as well as the basic features of other machines. As new machines are always coming on the market, I will post and update this information on my website.

Vibration Machines Comparisons

This information was accurate as of December 2019. See Becky's Vibrant Health website (www.BCVibrantHealth.com) for the latest updates.

Single-Motor Vertical (Linear) Vibration Machines (Recommended)

Vibrant Health: Currently two machines are available. The g-force for my machines is proprietary information, which is why I don't list amplitudes and g-forces. My machines are designed to heal, but exactly what goes into creating this vibration is complicated, and my formula is restricted. There are many factors that go into creating this best type of vibration; other companies cannot copy my machines, as they are not aware of what is needed. I am a world expert with twenty years' experience using whole body vibration with myself and others. My results (see appendix) and my books are your assurance that my machines will provide you with what you need. I cannot vouch for other companies' machines.

1. VIBRANT HEALTH POWER 1000: Vibrant Health's most popular model, this machine delivers a vibration powerful enough to give you an intense workout, but it is still gentle enough to be very safe and easy to use. This machine is designed for people of all ages. It is especially ideal for baby boomers and seniors who are facing the challenges of aging—aching joints, weight gain, bone loss, low energy, failing memory, mood swings, sleep problems, and many other age-related issues. It is the perfect machine for optimizing health—applicable to children, busy adults, and seniors. It will deliver a challenging workout and/or deep massage and stretching for tight muscles. Standing upright on this plate, you will feel the vibration travel through your entire body and up into your head—but don't worry, it feels good and is not bad for you!

The vertical vibration motion of this machine feels like a powerful cheetah purring. Because this motion is so smooth, the average person, with normal balance, will not need a handle to hold on to. If you do have balance issues, you can buy an optional tower and handle to go with the machine, use a separate balance bar, or put the vibration plate next to something else to hold on to. There are also two kinds of straps for use with different arm exercise positions: stretchy and non-stretchy.

Frequency range: 26–45 Hz
Cost: $999

2. VIBRANT HEALTH GENTLE 500: This machine provides the best type of vibration—but gentler. The amplitude of the motion is less than that of the Vibrant Health Power 1000, making this machine more suited to more fragile people.

When you stand on this vertical vibration machine, it produces a motion similar to a cat purring; you will feel the vibration travel up your body into your legs. You can get vibration into other parts of your body by sitting on the machine or doing exercises where your hands are on the machine, such as push-ups.

There is a tower with the control panel right in front of you and a handle to hold on to for people with balance issues.

This gentle machine is ideal for those on a budget or with age and/or health issues that make them more sensitive.

Frequency range: 30–45 Hz
Cost: $499

VibePlate: They have eight different models with different-sized plates, but all models have the same type of vibration.

Maximum amplitude: 2 mm
Frequency range: 10–60 Hz
Cost: ranges from $1,195 to $6,995

Bulletproof: There is only one model.

Maximum amplitude: 4 mm
Frequency: 30 Hz (no variability)
Cost: $1,495

Sonic Vibration Machines (Recommended)

SonicLife: There are four models of Sonix vibration machines.

Frequency ranges: 4–30 Hz for the least expensive model;
3–70 Hz for the most expensive model
Cost: ranges from $2,995 to $9,995

Double-Motor and Double-Motion Vibration Machines (NOT Recommended)

The motion is called by numerous different names, often reflecting complicated systems (in which more than one direction and type of movement can operate at the same time) and/or the very forceful nature of this type of machine: triplaner, spiral, circular, three-dimensional, horizontal, triangular, tri-phasic, multidimensional, omniflex, and piston. Double-motion machines will also include oscillation motion. Generally, for the triplaner type of motion, amplitudes range from 3–6 mm, frequencies ranges are 20–50 Hz, and maximum g-forces are 6–15 g. Oscillation motion modes have amplitudes of 1–12 mm, frequencies of 1–20 Hz, and maximum g-forces up to 8 g.

PowerPlate: There are eleven triplaner models.

Cost: ranges from $1,495 to $12,995

DKN: They have four triplaner models.

Cost: ranges from $2,499 to $4,699

Vmax: There are numerous different models (including Vmax, Pulser, Trio, ProDuo, Elite, Q2, Q5), most of which can run with both types of motion.

Cost: ranges from $1,248 to $4,699

IVibration: There is one model with multiple types of vibration produced concurrently.

Cost: $1,695

Tectonic: They have three models, two of which are double motion, and one is oscillation motion only.

Cost: ranges from $1,795 to $2,899

TriFlex: This is similar to some Vmax models, running with both types of motion, but is less expensive.

Oscillation Vibration Machines

This is the most popular type of machine (see the long list below of companies making and selling these machines), as you can achieve a high amplitude and g-force for a low price—but this does not mean it is the best type of vibration for you. Also known as pivotal, or teeter-totter, this type of motion can be destabilizing for joints and stressful for the mind and body. (See the earlier section about oscillation machines.) Some of these companies are actually selling the same machines, marketed under different names (notice how similar they look in pictures online). Amplitude ranges are usually 1–10 mm, frequency ranges are usually 1–20 Hz, and maximum g-forces can go up to 8 g. Prices can range from a few hundred dollars to three thousand dollars.

Bluefin
Body Trim Fitness
Confidence Fitness
Hurdle
HyperVibe
iDeer
LifePro
Maketec
Merax
Noblerex K1
Pinty
Rock Solid
T-Zone
VibraPro
Vmax
    (models Vmax i25 and Vmax Elite 300)
Zazz

Contraindications

It is always advisable to consult with your physician before starting any exercise program. Ongoing research in the field of whole body vibration indicates that many people can benefit from this form of exercise. However, if you suffer from any of the following contraindications, it is imperative that you discuss WBV therapy with your physician before beginning any training program with WBV equipment.

Please do not use any WBV device without first getting approval from your doctor if you have any of the following:

Relative contraindications—meaning that with special care and treatment, these conditions can sometimes not be a hindrance to, and may even benefit from, WBV.

- pregnancy
- epilepsy (very mild and not needing to be controlled with medications)
- minor migraines (mild, infrequent, and not needing to be controlled by medication)
- gallstones, kidney stones, bladder stones (WBV can help small stones move out of the body, but large ones may get stuck, potentially leading to severe problems.)
- articular rheumatism, arthrosis
- acute rheumatoid arthritis
- heart failure
- cardiac dysrhythmia
- cardiac disorders (post-myocardial infarction [heart attack])
- metal or synthetic implants (e.g., pacemaker, artificial cardiac valves, recent stents, or brain implants)
- chronic back pain (after fracture, disc disorders, or spondylosis)
- severe diabetes mellitus with peripheral vascular disease or neuropathy
- tumors (excluding metastases in the musculoskeletal system)

- spondylolisthesis without gliding
- movement disorders: Parkinson's disease, MS, cerebral palsy, and others
- chondromalacia of the joints of the lower extremities, osteonecrosis
- arterial circulation disorders
- venous insufficiency with ulcus cruris
- Morbus Sudeck Stadium II (or complex regional pain syndrome [CRPS])
- lymphatic edema
- postoperative wounds

Absolute contraindications—meaning *do not use* any WBV device at all if you have any of the following or if you have any concerns about your physical health! Note: conditions for which absolutely no vibration can be tolerated—such as broken bones, recent joint replacements and implants, and others—be aware that vibration will travel through wooden floors. In these cases, do not sit or stand next to a powerful vibrating plate. Cement floors are safe, as very little vibration will transmit through cement.

- acute inflammations, infections, and/or fever
- large gallstones, kidney stones, bladder stones (large enough to potentially get stuck in narrow tubes on the way out of your body)
- acute arthropathy or arthrosis
- joint replacements: You must wait six months after a joint replacement before using WBV. After that time, WBV is okay;

the vibration will then improve the bond of bone to metal or other synthetic material.

- bone fractures: For simple bone fractures, after six weeks it is okay to use WBV. For complex fractures or those involving implanted metal plates or screws, you must wait eight to twelve weeks before using WBV. Please consult with your doctor regarding your particular situation.

- acute migraine

- acute or severe epilepsy, (i.e., needs to be controlled with medication)

- retinal detachment (or a high risk of retinal detachment)

- fresh (surgical) wounds

- implants of the spine

- acute or chronic deep vein thrombosis or other thrombotic afflictions

- acute disc-related problems, spondylosis, gliding spondylolisthesis, or fractures

- severe osteoporosis with BMD less than 70 mg/ml (T-scores less than -3.9)

- spasticity (after stroke, spinal cord lesion, etc.)

- Morbus Sudeck Stadium I (CRPS I)

- tumors with metastases in the musculoskeletal system

- vertigo or positional dizziness

- acute myocardial infarction

CHAPTER 9

Getting Started and Physical Therapy

First in this chapter are daily plans for how to get started, a beginner's program, and guidelines for more advanced users. As stated before, WBV is an intensive workout, but, for most people, it won't make you feel sweaty and exhausted—so jump right in!

The second half of the chapter is devoted to using WBV for specific joint, muscle, and nerve issues. Research in the field of whole body vibration has shown that many people with joint, muscle, and nerve issues can benefit from this form of therapeutic exercise. However, if you suffer from any of these conditions, and before starting any therapeutic and/or exercise program. it is advisable to discuss WBV therapy with your physician.

Whole Body Vibration Training Basics

Goals

♦ Minimum recommended usage (but work up to this slowly): five to ten minutes of vibration at mid-level frequency each day, but it is not a problem if you miss some days. It is great if you can work up to doing twenty minutes per day.

♦ Maximum recommended usage: twenty to thirty minutes of vibration per day.

Basics

♦ To target different muscle groups, choose different positions from the pictures in this book or from the poster found on my website. The poster also shows the muscle groups each exercise position targets.

♦ Do each exercise position for thirty seconds to one minute, either holding the position (static, or isometric) or moving in and out of it (dynamic, or kinetic).

♦ Many benefits are achieved even if you only stand on the machine. In fact, standing upright on the plate is a great position for increasing bone density, as it helps to transmit the vibration throughout your body. So, even if you are too tired to work out, do stand or sit on your plate—relax and vibrate!

♦ Begin with the lowest speed (26Hz) to allow your body to adjust to vibration. Low speeds are also excellent for warming up and cooling down after exercise. Mid-level speed settings (30-38) are optimal for muscle-strengthening exercises, massage, and lymphatic drainage. Higher speed settings (upper 30s to 45) provide intense nervous system and brain stimulation.

Becky's Slow and Gentle Beginner's Program

DAY 1: Stand on your vibration machine (make sure you are using the proper type of machine) for thirty to sixty seconds at the lowest frequency or speed setting. WBV has very powerful effects on every part of your body, so I recommend starting with a very small amount of vibration on the first day to see how you respond. Watch and wait for twenty-four hours before trying any more vibration. As long as you feel the same or better the next day, you can increase the intensity of your next vibration session. *Some people will be able to increase the amount of WBV much faster than other people. If you find that you are feeling better following the beginner's program, you can try increasing your time and speed more rapidly.*

DAY 2: Increase the time by thirty to sixty seconds, staying at the same low speed. More sensitive people should do the same amount of time for two to three days before increasing, and increase the time by only thirty seconds each session thereafter.

EACH FOLLOWING DAY (or every two to three days): Increase the time by thirty to sixty seconds, up to ten minutes, *without increasing the speed.*

- ♦ When you get to ten minutes, drop the time down to three to four minutes and increase the speed one setting. Increase the time at this new speed following the same guidelines as above.

- ♦ As you gradually increase the speed, one setting at a time, follow this same pattern of increasing the amount of time day by day. Continue to drop the time back down when you increase the speed setting.

Troubleshooting

- ♦ If you feel worse in the twenty-four hours after your vibration session, try less time and/or frequency the next time. You can even rest a day and only vibrate two to three times per week. Another good way to slow down is to just sit next to the machine and put only your feet on the vibrating plate.

- ♦ It is common to experience itching in some areas of the body, such as ears, nose, or feet, while vibrating. This may be due to increased circulation in that area, a release of toxins, or possibly some energy phenomenon. While this itching can be irritating, as long as it stops shortly after vibrating, it is harmless—a minor inconvenience in the process of healing.

♦ It is also highly recommended to incorporate a healthy diet and natural supplements to help lower inflammation levels in your body. See the detoxification section in chapter 7 (pages 105–111) and the troubleshooting section in chapter 2 (pages 27–29).

Advanced Program

After you have acclimated to WBV and built up your tolerance and strength, you can maximize the health and wellness workout benefits by following these training tips.

Whole body vibration exercise is much more intense than conventional exercises. Workout times can be drastically shortened; you can accomplish the same results in ten minutes that would take you sixty minutes with conventional exercise. This is true because WBV requires your body to constantly respond to the rapidly moving platform beneath you.

Four factors determine how effective and challenging your training sessions are:

1. the frequency (rate of vibration)

2. the position or posture you assume

3. the amount of time you spend holding a given position

4. the amount of weight you are supporting on the plate (if you want a more challenging workout, hold additional exercise weights)

Static versus Dynamic Exercises

Exercises can be done statically or dynamically. Static exercises are more appropriate for beginners or when starting to rehabilitate from an injury. Dynamic exercises are great if you are looking to make an exercise more challenging.

- Static exercise: Holding a pose in a position without moving while the WBV machine is on
- Dynamic exercise: Moving while the WBV machine is on (e.g., doing push-ups or squats)

Progressive Training Plan

I recommend progressively phasing in the following elements to increase the difficulty of your workout. As your body adapts and grows stronger, you can continue to challenge yourself with these methods.

1. Extend the time of each exercise.
2. Reduce the rest period between exercises.
3. Increase the number of sets per exercise.
4. Perform exercise statically (standing still) then dynamically (moving).
5. Add more challenging exercises.
6. Increase the frequency (Hz).
7. Incorporate unilateral exercises (perform exercise on one leg).
8. Incorporate holding increasing amounts of additional weight.

See the color photos at the end of this chapter for sample exercise, massage, and stretching positions.

Using WBV as Physical Therapy

Ongoing research in the field of whole body vibration indicates that many people with joint, muscle, and nerve issues can benefit from this therapeutic system. However, if you suffer from any of the conditions mentioned below, or have unexplained or severe pain, please consult with your physician before beginning your WBV program.

The conditions discussed in the next pages are some of the most common musculoskeletal issues, not an exhaustive list of all possibilities. For a diagnosis of your condition, please see a physician.

If an injury or condition is chronic and not severe, start by standing on the plate, allowing the vibration to move throughout your whole body, promoting lower systemic inflammation.

Chronic conditions: If an injury or condition is chronic and not severe, start by standing on the plate, allowing the vibration to move throughout your whole body, promoting lower systemic inflammation. There is no need to stress an injured or inflamed joint by exercising at the beginning. Use massage and stretching positions as feels comfortable. See the exercise and massage positions in this book or on the exercise poster (see my website) for suggested positions to target your problem areas. Feel free to create your own stretches and massages.

A point to keep in mind: WBV should not be painful. It is okay if you are more aware of a particular area—if it feels different, tingly, stretched, or even uncomfortable. But when the sensation moves to significant pain, you are doing too much and should stop. Use common sense; a little discomfort that actually sort of feels good can be okay, but significant pain is your body telling you to "Stop!" In this case, try using less pressure (weight), time, and/or a lower frequency setting, or moving that part of the body away from the vibration. Later, when you have healed more, you can try more direct vibration on this part of your body again.

You should also use the appropriate amount of vibration for your overall health. So, if you have never done vibration before, and/ or your general health is not strong, you should follow the earlier guidelines for getting started. If your overall health is strong, or you have already been vibrating in the recent past, you will likely be able to use more vibration.

Acute injuries or conditions: For acute injuries that are not serious, such as strained or pulled muscles or tendons or minor sprains, you can try some vibration, but keep the affected part of the body off the vibrating plate if the vibration is painful. When pain levels are high, the key is to not allow vibration directly into an acutely injured and/or inflamed area of the body.

When pain levels are high, the key is to not allow vibration directly into an acutely injured and/ or inflamed area of the body.

Later, after inflammation levels have decreased enough so that you can use the affected joints and tissues without significant pain, move on to strengthening the muscle and tendons with exercises on the vibrating plate. This is an excellent way to increase the long-term health of your joints. Use the exercise chart available on my website to choose exercises that will target the muscles around the affected areas. The exercise chart is organized by muscle groups, areas of the body affected, and from beginner to advanced levels, so it is easy to choose appropriate exercises. Energy exercises—such as yoga, tai chi, tao, breathing exercises, and others—can also be very beneficial. Adapt as needed to do these safely while on the vibrating plate.

Common Conditions

Arthritis: WBV is very effective for osteoarthritis, the most common type of arthritis. I have had many people report great results with WBV for this relatively uncomplicated form of arthritis, which can affect joints anywhere in the body. See the guidelines in the next section for particular areas of discomfort.

> *After inflammation levels have decreased . . . , move on to strengthening the muscle and tendons with exercises on the vibrating plate.*

For autoimmune issues—such as rheumatoid arthritis, psoriatic arthritis, and other autoimmune diseases—or body-wide conditions, such as fibromyalgia, go slowly. Start by sitting next to the vibrating plate with only your feet on the plate. If you begin to feel worse, try resting a day or two, then starting up again with more caution. See also the troubleshooting section above.

Osteoporosis or Osteopenia: *When you want to increase bone density, it is important to get a strong vibrational signal to the entire* *body to improve all your bones*. Start by simply standing upright on the vibrating plate. In this position, on a machine with sufficient power, such as the Vibrant Health Power 1000, the vibration will travel from your feet all the way up to your head, missing only your arms and hands. Do additional positions, such as shoulder presses or push-up positions, to target these areas (see pages 164–165).

Adding in other exercise positions to increase muscle strength is also beneficial, as this will help protect you from falling. Slowly increase the amount of time you are vibrating, incorporating exercise positions as you go, to ten minutes of WBV a day. (See the exercise positions at the end of this chapter or on the exercise chart on Vibrant Health's website.)

Balance Issues: *Add a balance bar or a handle to your vibration machine to be sure you are safe on your plate.* The Vibrant Health Power 1000 machine has an optional tower with a handle to hold on to. The Vibrant Health Gentle 500 machine includes a control tower with handles. Other inexpensive options would be to hold on to a sturdy piece of furniture, exercise equipment, or nearby stair railing, or install a shower bar on the wall next to your vibration plate.

Holding on to your balance aid, stand and exercise on your vibration machine, slowly building up your time and frequency as outlined earlier in this chapter. As you are able, try some of the specific balance positions illustrated at the end of this chapter. However, *any* position in which your feet are on the plate will send a powerful signal through your nervous system, stimulating your proprioceptors, the parts that control balance.

Note that it is always okay to hold on to your balance aid when pre-forming any exercise or position on the vibration plate.

Lymphatic Drainage: Lymphatic drainage is a normal part of our detoxification or waste removal system. *Increasing lymphatic drainage is good for everyone, but in certain conditions, such as with lipedema and lymphedema, improving lymphatic drainage with WBV can be particularly helpful.*

All vibration is excellent for promoting increased lymphatic drainage, but when the legs are swollen, focusing on these areas can be especially helpful. Stand on your plate in positions 1 or 2, described at the end of the chapter, or sit next to the plate (position 4) if standing is too painful. You could also do leg massages, position 8 (see also other massages in the exercise section at the end of chapter). If your arms are also affected, use position 6 to get extra vibration into your arms. Gradually build up your time following the guidelines at the beginning of this chapter.

Physical Therapy by Body Area

The section below is organized by the area of the body where there is a problem, from toes to head. In my experience, having used WBV with hundreds of people with musculoskeletal and other mobility issues, where the problem is located and how severe it is are often the most important issues. Of lesser importance is exactly which type of inflammation you have; that is, arthritis, tendonitis, bursitis, neuropathy, overused muscles, or pulled tendons, ligaments, or muscles. Used gently, WBV can promote healing for many types of injuries. **Follow the guidelines in the first section of this chapter for length of time**

and frequency settings. For photos of the recommended positions, see the color section at the end of this chapter (pages 151–172).

FEET AND ANKLES

Chronic issues: Arthritis, gout, plantar fasciitis and other inflamed tendon issues, nerve issues such as peripheral neuropathy and Morton's neuromas, poor circulation, osteoporosis or osteopenia, old injuries not fully healed

Recommendation: Stand on the vibrating plate. If this is uncomfortable, try sitting next to the vibrating plate resting your feet on the plate. *Use positions 1, 2, or 4.* For autoimmune issues such as rheumatoid arthritis, use additional care—start by sitting next to the vibrating plate with only your feet on the plate.

Acute issues: Sprained ankles, pulled Achilles tendons, plantar fasciitis, and other strained tendons and muscles

Recommendation: Use a position designed to keep an injured foot, ankle, or leg off the vibration plate. *Use positions 3, 5, 6, or 7.* Ankle issues are often aggravated by vibration; you may find that you need to keep an injured ankle off the plate for quite a while. When vibration no longer aggravates your problem area, you can put your foot directly on the vibrating plate.

KNEES

Chronic issues: Arthritis, bursitis, tendonitis, osteoporosis or osteopenia, old injuries not fully healed, joint replacements older than six months

Recommendation: Stand on the vibrating plate or sit next to the vibrating plate while resting your feet on the plate. You can also massage and stretch your legs. *Use positions 1, 2, 4, or 8.*

Acute issues: Sprains and strains; torn meniscus, cartilage, or tendons

Recommendation: Start with positions that keep vibration out of your injured knee(s). *Use positions 3, 5, or 6.* When your doctor allows you to walk, you could try standing on the plate. If this is uncomfortable, go back to positions that keep the vibration out of your injured leg.

Hips

Chronic issues: Arthritis, bursitis, tendonitis, osteoporosis or osteopenia, old injuries not fully healed, joint replacements older than six months

Recommendation: Stand on the vibrating plate or sit next to the vibrating plate, resting your feet on the plate. If your hips and body can tolerate sitting directly on the plate without discomfort, you can also do this. *Use positions 1, 2, or 4 (as comfortable).*

Acute issues: Sprains, strains, torn cartilage

Recommendation: Start with positions that keep vibration out of your hips. *Use positions 4, 6, or 8.* When your doctor allows you to walk, you could try standing on the plate. If this is uncomfortable, go back to positions that keep the vibration out of your injured hip area.

BACK AND NECK

The back is a tricky area. Back issues are very common, and WBV is very effective for alleviating some of the most common causes of back pain; for example, tight muscles. Scientific research reports excellent results, especially for lower back pain.[1-4] Our own Vibrant Health survey results showed an average 45 percent drop in pain in back pain. Another common source of back pain is disk issues, and vibration is also good for *protecting* you from an acute episode of disk-related problems—but vibration should *not* be used when disk issues are already acute. Please check the contraindications (pages 128–131) for other back issues. As your neck is an extension of the spine, the same sorts of issues apply to the neck as well.

Chronic issues: Muscle tightness and soreness, arthritis, mild scoliosis (curvature of the spine), osteoporosis or osteopenia, old injuries not fully healed

Recommendation: For back pain that is not severe and not due to a contraindication, *using positions 1, 2, or 7* can potentially provide quick relief. Try standing on the plate, following the beginner guidelines in first part of this chapter, using positions 1 and 2. Note that the more you bend your knees, the less vibration gets into your back—adjust as needed. If you are quite limber and your back issue is only tight, sore muscles, you can try lying on your back on the plate for a back massage as described in position 7. If vibration directly into your back is aggravating your condition, you can try other positions that keep even more vibration out of your back.

Acute issues: Pulled or strained muscles or tendons, sciatica nerve pain

Recommendation: The sciatic nerves are large nerves, one on each side of the body, that exit the spinal column through several openings in the vertebrae and run down the legs. If either of these nerves is pinched by tight muscles, then WBV can provide quick effective relief; but if the nerve is pinched by bulging discs, then vibrating can make the problem worse. **Do not use WBV with a herniated or bulging disc.** If it is not a disk issue, still be extra careful and start with only thirty seconds. *Stand on the plate, using positions 1 or 2, following the guidelines for beginning and using WBV at start of this chapter. If standing on the plate aggravates your condition, try positions 4, 6, or 8.*

SHOULDERS

Chronic issues: Arthritis, rotator cuff tendonitis/impingement ("frozen shoulder"), bursitis, osteoporosis or osteopenia, old injuries not fully healed

Recommendation: Stand on the vibrating plate, ideally with your knees and legs straight so that vibration travels into your upper body. There is no need to directly place your shoulder on the plate. Putting your hands on the plate with weight on your hands (such as push-ups) to get more vibration into your shoulder will also put stress on your shoulder—only use these positions if they are comfortable for you. *Use positions 1, 5, 6, or 7.*

Acute issues: sprains, strains, torn cartilage, rotator cuff strains

Recommendation: Start with positions that do not allow vibration into your shoulders. *Use positions 2, 4, or 8.* When your doctor says that it is okay to use your shoulder, you could try standing on the plate. If this is uncomfortable, stop and go back to the positions that keep the vibration out of the injured area.

Hands, Wrists, and Elbows

Chronic issues: Arthritis, tennis elbow, carpal tunnel syndrome, writer's cramp, tingling or numbness, poor circulation, trigger finger, repetitive motion syndrome, bursitis, osteoporosis or osteopenia, old injuries not fully healed

Recommendation: If it is not uncomfortable for you, you can place your hands on the plate for direct vibration into the hands and arms. Do not put weight on your hands if this is painful. Stretch your fingers as is comfortable, or relax and allow the vibration to massage your hands and arms. If direct vibration into your hands and arms is uncomfortable, any other position will get vibration into your body and may help. If otherwise comfortable, you can stand, sit, or lie on the vibrating plate. *Try to use position 6 first; if that is painful, you can use any other position that is comfortable.*

Acute issues: sprains, strains

Recommendation: Start with positions that do not allow vibration into your hands and arms. *Use positions 1, 2, 4, 5, or 8.* When you can use your hands, you could try placing them on the plate. If this is uncomfortable, stop and go back to the positions that keep the vibration out of the injured area.

Head

Chronic and Acute: Headaches, memory problems, depression, anxiety, movement and nerve problems, neurological diseases

Headaches: Headaches that are not migraines are often helped by vibration; for example, stress or tension headaches and/or headaches due to tight muscles are likely to improve, as vibration is an excellent stress reducer and muscle massager/relaxer. You can try standing with your legs straight—this will help tight muscles in your back, neck, and shoulders—or with your legs bent, if vibration in your head bothers you. Sit next to the machine in a chair if the headache is severe. Any position that is comfortable for you is good—it is all about relaxing! *Use positions 1–8, as long as you are comfortable.*

There have been reports of mild migraines improving—that is, the number and intensity decreasing—with very small amounts of *gentle vibration applied when you do not have a migraine.* **Try this only when you do not actually have or expect a migraine.** Use caution—start with just thirty seconds sitting next to the plate with only your feet on the plate. Do not try any vibration with severe or frequent migraines or those that must be controlled with medications.

Mood and/or neurological system and movement issues: Any position that is comfortable, safe, and secure for you will be fine. Having any body part on the vibrating plate will automatically cause large numbers of neurons to fire signals into your brain at the same rate the machine is vibrating, twenty to fifty times per second. This is a massive neurological stimulation, lighting your brain up and inducing it to release neurotransmitters that will almost immediately help your brain function better, leading to improved sleep, energy, and mood. Longer term, the stimulation will help your neurons grow stronger and thicker and make new connections to other neurons in your brain, aiding in learning. If you can tolerate standing on the plate, that will give you greater brain stimulation, as will building up your time on the plate. These are good goals to work toward but going slowly is best. *Use positions 1–8, as is comfortable and safe for you.*

With careful use of WBV, you can promote healing and lower pain and inflammation levels for numerous chronic issues. But many of these issues can flare up at times and become more acute. Use caution (go more slowly) at these times.

Good luck, be patient, and enjoy!!

Physical Therapy Positions

These positions are recommended for isolating vibration to particular body areas. Use these positions with the preceding physical therapy recommendations (pages 142–149).

Standing Positions

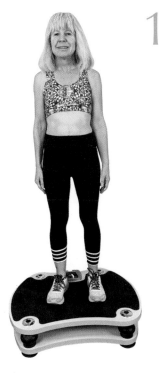

1

Standing straight: Stand on the plate with your legs completely straight. *This position will cause the vibration to transmit through your bones up into your entire body (except for your arms and hands).*

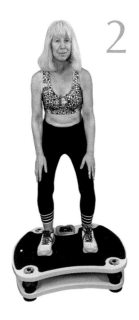

2

Standing with knees bent: Stand on the plate with your knees bent. Notice that when you bend your knees, the vibration immediately moves out of your upper body. If you do not like the sensation of vibration in your head, bend your knees. The more you bend your knees, the harder your legs will work in this position. Be sure to keep your knees lined up vertically with your toes—not beyond your toes—as this will put too much pressure on the knees. To go lower, push your rear end out behind you (as if you were going to sit down on a chair). *This position keeps most of the vibration in your legs.*

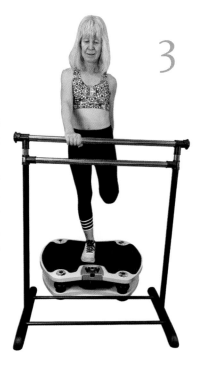

3

Standing on one leg: Use a balance bar or other balancing aid so that you can safely stand on one foot. (Inexpensive options would be to hold onto another sturdy piece of furniture, exercise equipment, nearby stair railing, or install a shower bar on the wall next to your vibration plate. You can hold your foot off the plate with one hand while holding on to the balancing aid with the other hand or use two hands on the balancing aid and hold your foot up with your leg muscles.

Sitting Positions

Feet only: Sit in a chair next to the machine and put just your feet on the machine. *This position will keep the vibration in only your feet and legs.*

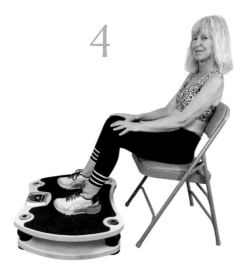

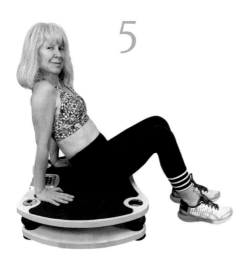

Sitting on plate: Sit on the plate, keeping your feet on the floor. You can rest your hands on the plate or sit up straight and keep your hands off the plate. *This position will keep the vibration in your upper legs, torso, and upper body.*

6

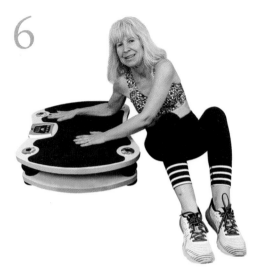

Arms only: Sit next to the plate and rest your hands and/or arms on the plate. *Vibration will only be in your arms, hands, and shoulders.*

Lying Down Positions

7

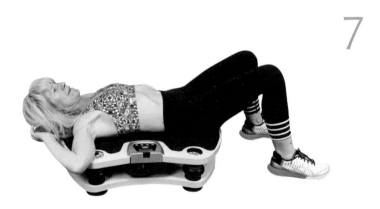

Back massage: If you are agile, you can lie on your back on the vibration plate, but be sure your head is not directly on the plate. Use thick padding or your hands to old your head off the plate. Your feet can rest on the floor or be held above you. *This position can be an effective back massage at the same time as keeping vibration out of your feet and lower legs.*

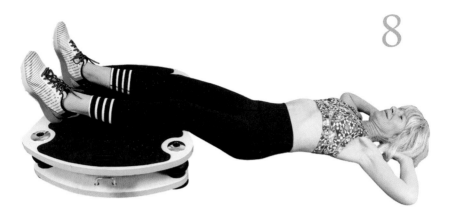

Calf massage: Lie on the floor and rest your calves on the vibration plate. *This position delivers a relaxing calf massage with little to no vibration getting into your upper body.*

Sample Exercise Positions, Massages, and Stretches

There are as many positions possible on the vibration plate as you can think of. Anything is fine; experiment and see what feels good. The muscle-strengthening effect is greatest when using exercise positions, but even if you just stand on the vibrating plate, you will still be getting many benefits. The exercises are grouped by the areas of your body you might wish to target, but many of these exercises will also be using muscles all over your body. Some positions work on one side of the body at a time; when you do these, to keep things even, you should switch sides and do the position on the other side, too. For pictures of more suggested positions, check my website at www.BCVibrantHealth.com.

For static exercises, you get into a position and hold it. For more intensive dynamic exercises, you can move slowly in and out of the position.

Leg, Hip, and Buttock Exercises

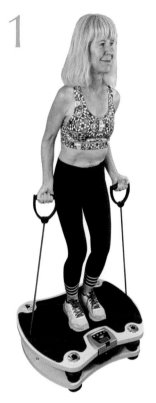

Beginner's position: Stand in a comfortable, balanced position with knees slightly flexed. If you enjoy the sensation of the vibration, you can straighten your legs, and more vibration will travel up through your bones to your entire body. If you don't like the vibration in your head, keep your knees bent. Hold onto the straps as desired.

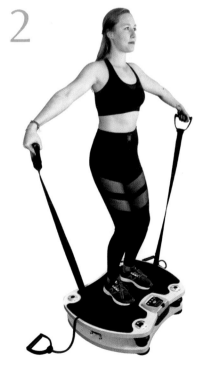

Squat with arms: Stand on the platform with legs slightly apart and in a slight squat. Holding onto the straps, stretch your arms out to the sides, palms down. Pull up on the straps.

3

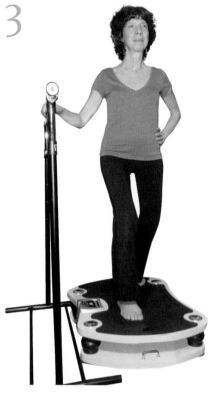

Walking position with squat: Place one foot in front of the other on the platform as if you were walking. Bend both knees. Hold a balance aid if needed.

4

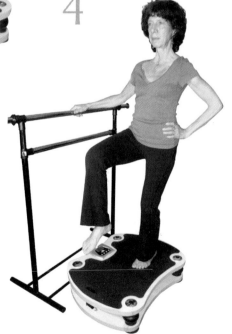

Single leg lift: Stand in the middle of the platform. Lift and hold one leg up in front of you so that your thigh is horizontal to the plate. Bend your knee to ninety degrees. Hold on to a balance aid as necessary.

Deep squat: Position your feet in the middle of the plate, slightly apart. Bend your knees about eighty degrees. Don't let your knees extend beyond your toes. Arch your back, keep your head up, and maintain balance. This position feels sort of like beginning to sit in a chair, then holding that position.

5

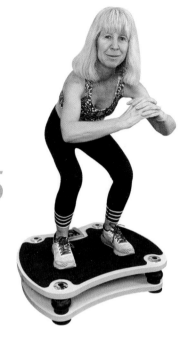

6

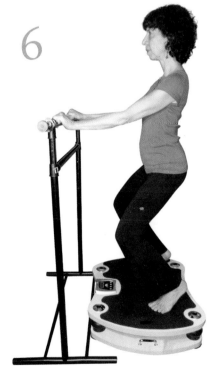

Calf exercise: Stand on the plate on your toes. Keep your knees slightly bent, back straight, and head up. Hold a balance aid as needed.

7

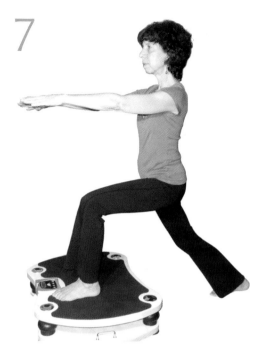

Lunge: Place one foot on the center of the platform. Extend the opposite foot backwards to the floor, bending the knee to make the exercise more difficult. Extend your arms straight out in front of you, or hold on to a balance aid as needed. Don't let your front knee extend beyond your toes. Keep your back straight and head up.

8

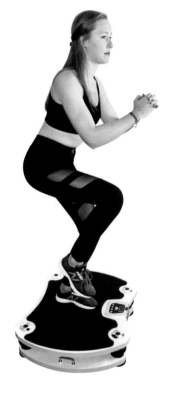

One-legged squat: Stand in the middle of the platform. Bend your knees and lift one foot up. Do not let your knee extend past your toes. Hold on to a balance aid as needed.

9

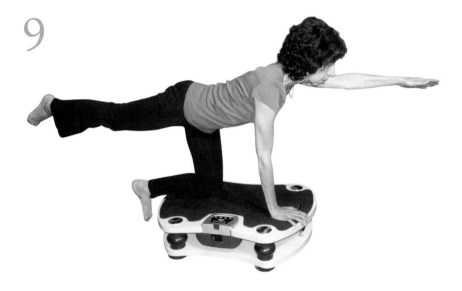

Superman pose: Place one knee and the opposite hand on the platform; rest your knee on a cushion or towel as needed. Raise and extend the opposite hand and leg. Raise your head, balance, and hold.

Arm, Chest, and Shoulder Exercises

10

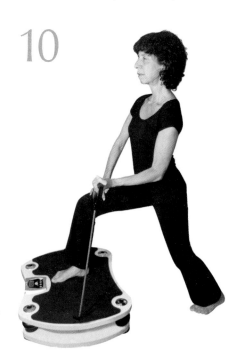

One-arm pull: Place one foot on the platform and keep the other foot on the ground behind you. Place the hand opposite the leg on the platform on that leg to brace yourself. Hold the stretchy strap in the other hand and, with your elbow bent, pull up.

11

Arm exercise with straps 1: Stand upright on the platform and, with arms stretched out to the sides and palms facing down, pull up on the cloth straps.

12

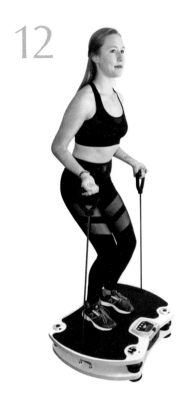

Arm exercise with straps 2: Stand on the plate with knees bent. Holding the adjustable straps, extend your arms in front of you palms up, elbows bent. Pull up on the straps.

13

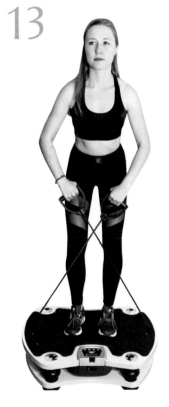

Crossed-strap pull: Stand on the plate in a slight squat. Hold each stretchy strap in the hand opposite to the side the strap is on and pull out to the side with elbows bent.

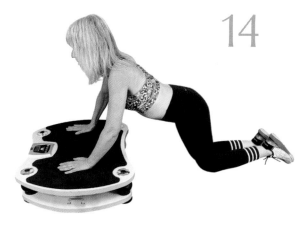

14

Beginner's push-up: Facing the plate, put your hands flat on the outer edges and keep your knees on the ground behind the plate. Line up your shoulders over your hands and pull in your stomach. You can either bend at your hips or, to make the exercise more difficult, drop your hips to make a straight line from shoulders to knees. Bend your elbows to hold your weight. The more you bend your elbows, the harder this exercise will be.

15

Advanced push-up: Facing the plate, put your hands flat on the outer edges and keep your feet on the ground behind the plate. Keep your back straight, shoulders over your hands, and stomach in. Bending and straightening your elbows, move up and down, doing push-ups; or just bend your elbows and hold that position.

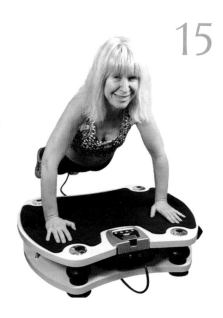

Shoulder press: Place your hands on the platform, fingers pointing forward. Align your shoulders above your hands. With your feet separated but close to the plate, stand on your toes if you can. To make this exercise more difficult, bend your elbows. This will increase the weight your arms and shoulders are supporting.

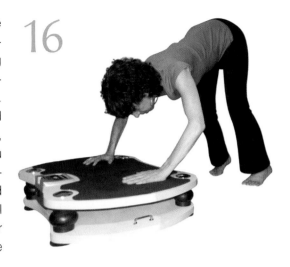

Triceps dip: With your back to the plate, place your hands at the front of the plate, shoulder width apart, pointing forward. Keeping your heels on the ground, bend your knees ninety degrees. Hold your waist in, keep your back straight and your head up. Lower your buttocks by bending your elbows and either hold that position or move up and down.

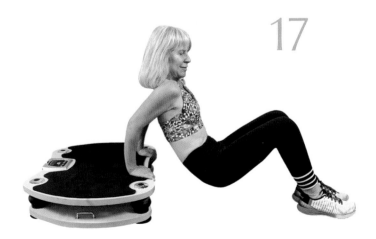

Abdominal and Core Exercises

18

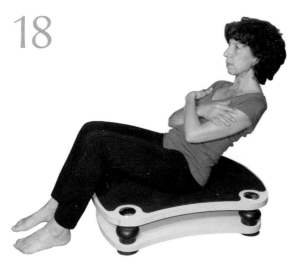

Easy abdominal 1: Sit on the platform with your feet on the floor. Lean back about forty-five degrees and cross your arms over your chest. Hold this position.

19

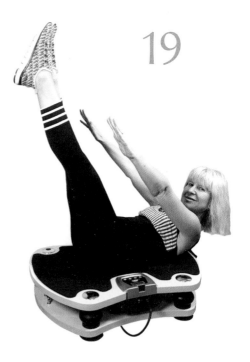

Easy abdominal 2: Lie on your back on the plate with both legs straight and pointing up. Stretch your arms straight out and up. Lift your head and shoulders up as high as you can. Do not allow your head to rest on the plate.

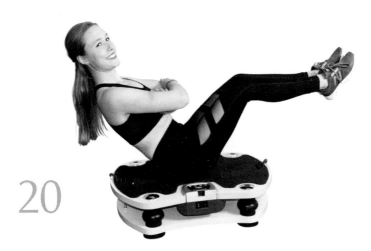

Advanced abdominal: Sit sideways on the plate in a V-shaped position, leaning back and lifting your legs. The straighter the legs in this position, the harder it will be. Try it with bent knees at first. This exercise targets abdominal muscles, which are essential for good posture and helping to prevent lower back pain.

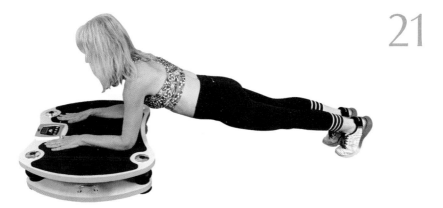

Plank: Position yourself face down with your forearms on the platform and your toes on the floor. Your elbows should be directly under your shoulders, and your hands should face forward. Keep your head relaxed. Tighten your abdominal muscles. Keep your back straight and your body in a straight line from ears to toes—no sagging or bending.

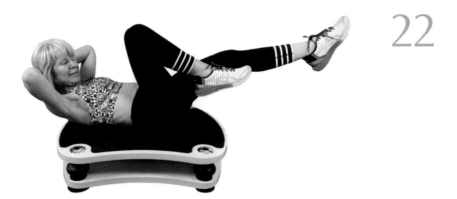

22

Easy diagonal crunch: Lie on your back on the platform. Lift your legs and bend one knee while straightening the other leg. Lift your head with your hands behind your head. Bring your opposite elbow to the bent knee if you can and hold while tensing your abdominal muscles.

23

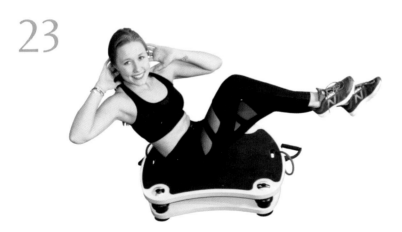

Advanced diagonal crunch: Sit lengthwise on the platform, leaning back and lifting your legs. Bend one knee while straightening the other leg. Bring your hands to ears and bend your elbows. Touch your opposite elbow to the bent knee and hold while tensing your abdominal muscles.

Balancing, Stretching, and Massage Positions

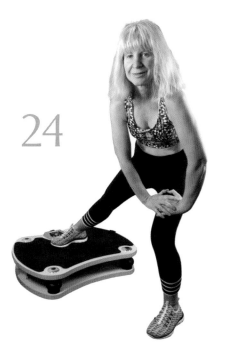

Adductor stretch: Stand in front of the plate, facing sideways. Place one foot on the plate, toward the back of the plate, so that your leg is stretched. With your weight on the leg on the floor, bend that knee and rest both hands on that knee. Slowly tense the inner thigh of the leg on the plate. This position stretches the muscles of your inner thigh.

24

25

One-leg balancing: Stand upright with your arms stretched straight out to the sides. Lift one leg off the plate and to the rear. Hold on to a balance aid as needed.

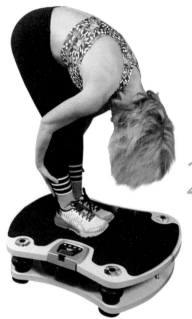

Hamstring stretch: Stand on the center of the plate with your feet together, knees slightly bent. Bend at the waist and grasp your ankles.

26

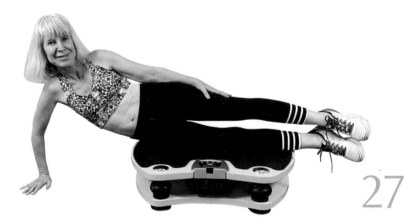

27

Abductor massage: Lie lengthwise on the plate with the side of your leg and buttocks resting on the plate. Place one hand on the floor for balance and to support your upper-body weight. Switch sides to massage the other leg.

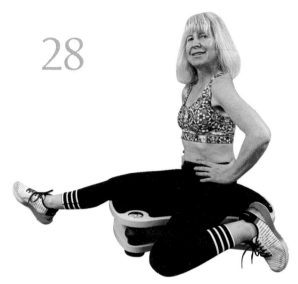

28

Hamstring massage: Sit on the plate with one leg stretched out straight and one leg bent and resting off the plate. Sit up straight but relaxed.

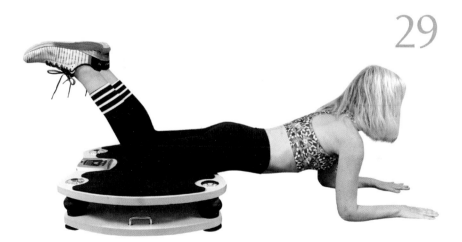

29

Quadriceps massage: Lie face down with your knees bent and your thighs on the plate. Support your body weight with your forearms and flatten your back. Look forward.

30

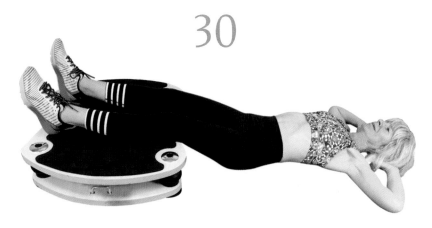

Calf massage: Place your calves on the plate, lie back on floor behind you, hands behind your head, and relax. This is a favorite position for many people.

After Whole Body Vibration

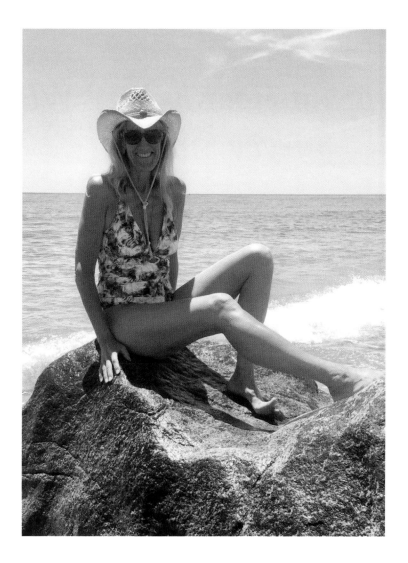

Becky Chambers, age 59

Vibrant Health 2019 WBV Survey Summary

Effects of Whole Body Vibration Using the Vibrant Health Power 1000 in Retrospective Observational Survey[x]

Becky Chambers, BS, MEd.,
and Jaswant Chaddha, MD, FACOG
(unpublished data, 2019)

Survey of People Who Use the Vibrant Health Power 1000 Machine

Specifications of the VH Power 1000 and method of use:

♦ Type of vibration machine: Relatively gentle, single moter, vertical vibration (entire plate moves in the same direction, up and down, at the same time)

♦ Frequency = 26–45 Hz (increasing in 1 Hz increments)

♦ Becky Chambers's "Slow & Gentle" method

---

[x]Becky Chambers and Jaswant Chaddha, "Effects of Whole Body Vibration Using the Vibrant Health Power 1000 in Retrospective Observational Survey," 2019, https://bcvibranthealth.com/wp-content/uploads/2019/06/Vibrant-Health-WBV-Survey2019.pdf.

Metrics of Study Respondents

- 53 respondents out of 187 surveys sent out using HIPPA-protected online Survey Monkey website (28% response rate) in two weeks; no compensation was offered.

- 26% were 50–59 years of age, 62% were age 60–80, 2% were over 90 years of age. A total of 90% of respondents were over age 50.

- 58% female, 42% male

- 80% in average, good, or excellent health (self-rating)

- Most reported eating a healthy diet and taking few to no drugs.

- 55% of the respondents had had their machine one to two years, 43% for one to twelve months.

- Most had never used a vibration machine before.

- 64% reported following Becky's "Slow & Gentle" plan for starting WBV; 54% said this approach was important to them.

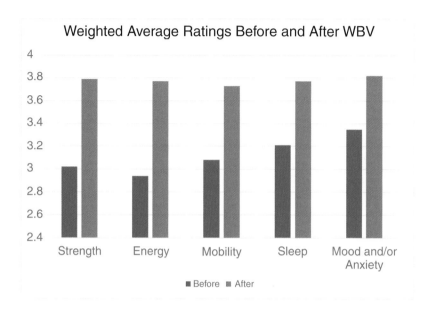

Weighted Average Ratings Before and After WBV

Five modalities—strength, energy, mobility, sleep, and mood/anxiety—were self-rated on a scale of 1 to 5, with "1" being weak/low/poor and "5" being very strong/high or excellent. Significant improvements were seen in strength, energy, mobility, sleep, and mood (25, 28, 20, 17, and 14 percent, respectively).

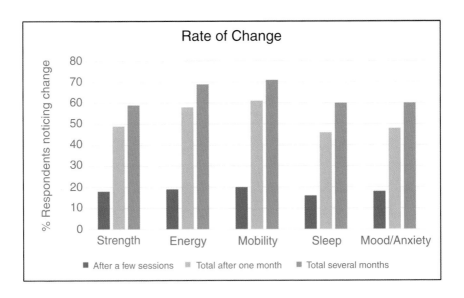

All modalities improved rapidly: strength, energy, mobility, sleep, and mood/anxiety.

- ◆ 15–20% improved after a few WBV sessions
- ◆ 45–60% total within a month
- ◆ 60–70% total within several months

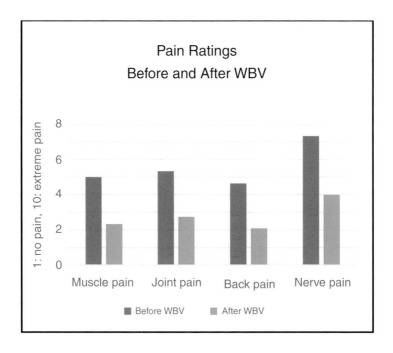

Thirty-nine respondents reported having muscle, joint, back, or nerve pain when they started vibrating. Of these respondents, 74 percent reported an average drop in pain levels of 52 percent within a few months of beginning WBV. Twenty percent of the thirty-nine respondents also reduced their pain medications after beginning WBV or switched to less powerful meds while reporting less pain. Most respondents took no pain medications.

Respondent comments:

"I am recovering/reversing from neuropathy. The WBV brought immediate results."

"My best results—a major decrease in sciatic pain!"

"I feel like my body and muscles are more flexible."

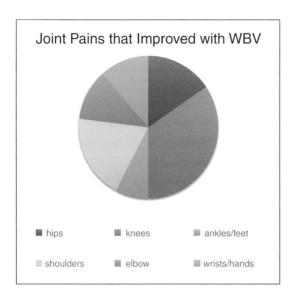

Joints all over the body improved, especially knee joints.

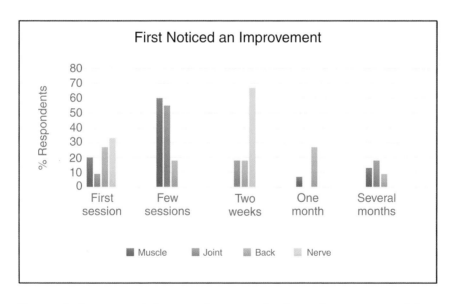

Pain relief was rapid for muscle, joint, back, and nerve pain. Most people whose pain improved noticed this improvement within weeks of beginning their WBV program.

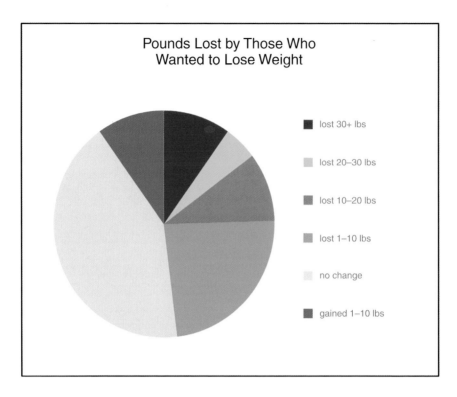

Pounds Lost by Those Who Wanted to Lose Weight

- lost 30+ lbs
- lost 20–30 lbs
- lost 10–20 lbs
- lost 1–10 lbs
- no change
- gained 1–10 lbs

Almost half of those who wanted to lose weight did lose weight, ranging from a few pounds to over thirty pounds. Virtually all of the respondents (98 percent) were not taking weight-loss supplements or medications. Most followed healthy, low carb diet regimes, and 86 percent did not change their diets. There was very little change in the amount or type of other exercise for most respondents.

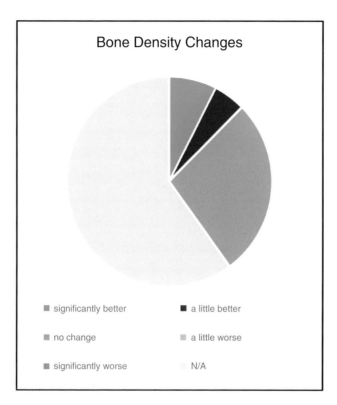

Bone density:

♦ 40% of respondents increased their bone density or did not lose bone density.

♦ 0% of respondents lost bone density.

♦ Considering that a large percentage of the respondents in this survey either already had osteopenia or osteoporosis, or were at high risk of developing low bone density, these results are excellent, indicating a reversal or interruption of the normal progression of this disease for 40% or more of the survey respondents.

♦ 60% answered Not Applicable (N/A): Most likely, many respondents had not used their machines long enough to have had a recent bone-density test and, therefore, were not able to answer to this question.

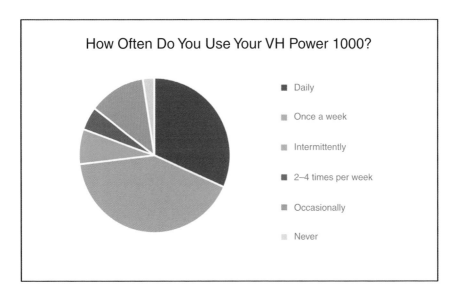

How Often Do You Use Your VH Power 1000?

- Daily
- Once a week
- Intermittently
- 2–4 times per week
- Occasionally
- Never

Seventy-three percent of respondents use their vibration machine at least two to four times per week. Only 8 percent use their machine occasionally or never.

Respondent comments:

"Great investment—really helps me, and my grandkids love it, too!"

"I really recommend its use to improve your health and quality of life."

"The most obvious response I have experienced is increased energy!"

"Exercise/mobility is vital to quality of life. I want to live, not just exist."

"This machine is the missing piece to my health recovery."

"It is the easiest thing to do and get results."

"Love it!"

"I love the muscle strength and increased mood it has provided."

"I feel that it was a wise investment."

"Noticed an increase in my upper-body muscle development."

"I love the gentle, deep massage feeling the machine provides. It is very relaxing, and I love doing qigong on my platform."

"Love it. I like to do the exercises on it."

"Great product. My girlfriend and I use it for five minutes twice a day while brushing our teeth. :)"

ENDNOTES

Chapter 1

1. D. J. Cochrane, "Vibration Exercise: The Potential Benefits," *International Journal of Sports Medicine* 32, no. 2 (2011): 75–99, doi:10.1055/s-0030-1268010.

2. R. W. Lau et al., "The Effects of Whole Body Vibration Therapy on Bone Mineral Density and Leg Muscle Strength in Older Adults: A Systematic Review and Meta-Analysis," *Clinical Rehabilitation* 25, no. 11 (November 2011): 975–88, doi:10.1177/0269215511405078.

3. H. Bokaeian, A. H. Bakhtiary, et al., "The Effect of Adding Whole Body Vibration Training to Strengthening Training in the Treatment of Knee Osteoarthritis: A Randomized Clinical Trial," *Journal of Bodywork and Movement Therapies* 20, no. 2 (April 2016), doi:10.1016/j.jbmt.2015.08.005.

4. T. Trans, J. Aaboe, M. Henriksen, R. Christensen, et al., "Effect of Whole Body Vibration Exercise on Muscle Strength and Proprioception in Females with Knee Osteoarthritis," *Knee* 16, no. 4 (August 2009): 256–61, doi:10.1016/j.knee.2008.11.014.

5. T. Tsuji, J. Yoon, T. Aiba, A. Kanamori, et al., "Effects of Whole-Body Vibration Exercise on Muscular Strength and Power, Functional Mobility and Self-Reported Knee Function in Middle-Aged and Older Japanese Women with Knee Pain. *Knee* 21, no. 6 (December 2014): 1088–95, doi:10.1016/j.knee.2014.07.015.

6. M. Roelants, C. Delecluse, S. M. Verschueren, "Whole-Body-Vibration Training Increases Knee-Extension Strength and Speed of Movement in Older Women," *Journal of the American Geriatrics Society* 52, no. 6 (June 2004): 901–8.

7. Y. G. Park, B. S. Kwon, J. W. Park, et al., "Therapeutic Effect of Whole Body Vibration on Chronic Knee Osteoarthritis," *Annals of Rehabilitation Medicine* 37, no. 4 (August 2013): 505–15, doi:10.5535/arm.2013.37.4.505.

8. N. A. Segal, N. A. Glass, N. Shakoor, and R. Wallace, "Vibration Platform Training in Women at Risk for Symptomatic Knee Osteoarthritis," *PM & R* 5, no. 3 (March 2013): 201–9, quiz 209, doi:10.1016/j.pmrj.2012.07.011.

9. S. Anwer, A. Alghadir, H. Zafar, and E. Al-Eisaaa, "Effect of Whole Body Vibration Training on Quadriceps Muscle Strength in Individuals with Knee Osteoarthritis: A Systematic Review and Meta-Analysis," *Physiotherapy* 102, no. 2 (June 2016): 145–151.

10. Becky Chambers and Jaswant Chaddha, "Effects of Whole Body Vibration Using the Vibrant Health Power 1000 in Retrospective Observational Survey," online document (2016), https://bcvibranthealth.com/wp-content/uploads /2019/06/Vibrant-Health-WBV-Survey2019.pdf.

Chapter 2

1. M. Zago, P. Capodaglio, C. Ferrario, et al., "Whole-Body Vibration Training in Obese Subjects: A Systematic Review," *PLoS One* 13, no. 9 (September 2018): e0202866, doi:10.1371/journal.pone.0202866.

2. C. Bosco et al., "Hormonal Responses to Whole-Body Vibration in Men," *European Journal of Applied Physiology* 81 (2000): 449–454.

3. Gina Kolata, "Low Buzz May Give Mice Better Bones and Less Fat." *New York Times* 30 (October 30, 2007), https://www.nytimes.com/2007/10/30/health /research/30bone.html?_r=1.

4. I. Janssen and R. Ross, "Effects of Sex on the Change in Visceral, Subcutaneous Adipose Tissue and Skeletal Muscle in Response to Weight Loss," *International Journal of Obesity and Related Metabolic Disorders* 23, no. 10 (1999): 1035–1046.

5. F. Yang, J. Munoz, L. zhu Han, and F. Yang, "Effects of Vibration Training in Reducing Risk of Slip-Related Falls among Young Adults with Obesity," *Journal of Biomechanics* 57 (May 2017): 87–93, doi:10.1016/j.jbiomech.2017. 03.024.

6. A. Figueroa, R. Kalfon, T. A. Madzima, and A. Wong, "Effects of Whole-Body Vibration Exercise Training on Aortic Wave Reflection and Muscle Strength in Postmenopausal Women with Prehypertension and Hypertension," *Journal of Human Hypertension* 28, no. 2 (February 2014): 118–122, doi:10.1038/jhh.2013.59.

7. A. Wong, S. Alvarez-Alvarado, A. W. Kinsey, and A. Figueroa, "Whole-Body Vibration Exercise Therapy Improves Cardiac Autonomic Function and Blood Pressure in Obese Pre- and Stage 1 Hypertensive Postmenopausal Women," *Journal of Alternative and Complementary Medicine* 22, no. 12 (2016): 970–976, doi:10.1089/acm.2016.0124.

8. A. Wong, S. Alvarez-Alvarado, S. J. Jaime, et al., "Combined Whole Body Vibration Training and L-Citrulline Supplementation Improves Pressure Wave Reflection in Obese Postmenopausal Women," *Applied Physiology, Nutrition, and Metabolism* 41, no. 3 (2016): 292–7, doi:10.1139/apnm-2015-0465.

9. B. Wilms, J. Frick, B. Ernst, et al., "Whole Body Vibration Added to Endurance Training in Obese Women: A Pilot Study," *International Journal of Sports Medicine* 33, no. 9 (2012): 740–743, doi:10.1055/s-0032-1306284.

10. G. Severino, M. Sanchez-Gonzalez, M. Walters-Edwards, et al., "Whole-Body Vibration Training Improves Heart Rate Variability and Body Fat Percentage in Obese Hispanic Postmenopausal Women," *Journal of Aging and Physical Activity* 25, no. 3 (July 2017): 395–401, doi:10.1123/japa.2016-0087.

11. C. Milanese, F. Piscitelli, M. G. Zenti, et al., "Ten-Week Whole-Body Vibration Training Improves Body Composition and Muscle Strength in Obese Women," *International Journal of Medical Sciences* 10, no. 3 (2013): 307–311, doi:10.7150/ijms.5161.

12. R. So, M. Eto, T. Tsujimoto, and K. Tanaka, "Acceleration Training for Improving Physical Fitness and Weight Loss in Obese Women," *Obesity Research and Clinical Practice* 8, no. 3 (May–June 2014): e201–e98, doi:10.1016/j.orcp.2013.03.002.

13. S. Alvarez-Alvarado, S. J. Jaime, M. J. Ormsbee, et al., "Benefits of Whole-Body Vibration Training on Arterial Function and Muscle Strength in Young Overweight/Obese Women," *Hypertension Research* 40, no. 5 (2017): 487–492, doi:10.1038/hr.2016.178.

14. A. Figueroa, R. Gil, A. Wong, et al., "Whole-Body Vibration Training Reduces Arterial Stiffness, Blood Pressure, and Sympathovagal Balance in Young Overweight/Obese Women," *Hypertension Research* 35, no. 6 (2012): 667–672, doi:10.1038/hr.2012.15.

15. M. E. Zaki, "Effects of Whole Body Vibration and Resistance Training on Bone Mineral Density and Anthropometry in Obese Postmenopausal Women," *Journal of Osteoporosis* (2014): 702589, doi:10.1155/2014/702589.

16. D. Vissers, A. Verrijken, I. Mertens, et al., "Effect of Long-Term Whole Body Vibration Training on Visceral Adipose Tissue: A Preliminary Report," *Obesity Facts* 3, no. 2 (2010): 93–100, doi:10.1159/000301785.

17. A. Figueroa, S. Alvarez-Alvarado, M. J. Ormsbee, et al., "Impact of L-Citrulline Supplementation and Whole-Body Vibration Training on Arterial Stiffness and Leg Muscle Function in Obese Postmenopausal Women with High Blood Pressure," *Experimental Gerontology* 63 (March 2015): 35–40, doi:10.1016/j .exger.2015.01.046.

18. A. Miyaki, S. Maeda, Y. Choi, et al., "The Addition of Whole-Body Vibration to a Lifestyle Modification on Arterial Stiffness in Overweight and Obese Women," *Artery Research* 6, no. 2 (June 2012): 85–91, doi:10.1016/j .artres.2012.01.006.

19. J. Adsuar, B. Del Pozo-Cruz, J. Parraca, et al., "Vibratory Exercise Training Effects on Weight in Sedentary Women with Fibromyalgia," *International Journal of Medicine and Science in Physical Education and Sport* 13 (2013): 295–305.

20. B. Sañudo, R. Alfonso-Rosa, B. Del Pozo-Cruz, et al., "Whole Body Vibration Training Improves Leg Blood Flow and Adiposity in Patients with Type 2 Diabetes Mellitus," *European Journal of Applied Physiology* 113, no. 9 (2013): 2245–2252, doi:10.1007/s00421-013-2654-3.

21. A. Bellia, M. Sallì, M. Lombardo, et al., "Effects of Whole Body Vibration Plus Diet on Insulin-Resistance in Middle-Aged Obese Subjects," *International Journal of Sports Medicine* 35, no. 6 (2014): 511–516, doi:10.1055/s-0033-1354358.

22. Zago et al., "Whole-Body Vibration Training in Obese Subjects."

23. Milanese et al., "Ten-Week Whole-Body Vibration Training."

24. Zaki, "Effects of Whole Body Vibration and Resistance Training."

25. Vissers et al., "Effect of Long-Term Whole Body Vibration Training."

26. Miyaki et al., "The Addition of Whole-Body Vibration to a Lifestyle Modification."

27. Adsuar et al., "Vibratory Exercise Training Effects on Weight."

28. Sañudo et al., "Whole Body Vibration Training Improves Leg Blood Flow."

29. Bellia et al., "Effects of Whole Body Vibration Plus Diet."

30. Vissers et al., "Effect of Long-Term Whole Body Vibration Training."

31. Wilms et al., "Whole Body Vibration Added to Endurance Training."

32. Severino et al., "Whole-Body Vibration Training Improves Heart Rate."

33. Milanese et al., "Ten-Week Whole-Body Vibration Training."

34. So et al., "Acceleration Training."

35. Figueroa et al., "Impact of L-Citrulline Supplementation."

36. Miyaki et al., "The Addition of Whole-Body Vibration to a Lifestyle Modification."

37. Sañudo et al., "Whole Body Vibration Training Improves Leg Blood Flow."

38. Miyaki et al., "The Addition of Whole-Body Vibration to a Lifestyle Modification."

39. Janssen and Ross, "Effects of Sex."

40. Wong et al., "Whole-Body Vibration Exercise Therapy."

41. Alvarez-Alvarado et al., "Benefits of Whole-Body Vibration Training."

42. Figueroa et al., "Whole-Body Vibration Training Reduces Arterial Stiffness."

43. Miyaki et al., "The Addition of Whole-Body Vibration to a Lifestyle Modification."

44. Ibid.

45. Yang et al., "Effects of Vibration Training."

46. Miyaki et al., "The Addition of Whole-Body Vibration to a Lifestyle Modification."

47. Wilms et al., "Whole Body Vibration Added to Endurance Training."

48. Bellia et al., "Effects of Whole Body Vibration Plus Diet."

49. Meghan McGee-Lawrence, K. H. Wenger, S. Misra, et al., "Whole-Body Vibration Mimics the Metabolic Effects of Exercise in Male Leptin Receptor-Deficient Mice," *Endocrinology* 158, no. 5 (2017):1160–1171, doi:10.1210/en.2016-1250.

50. H. Yin, H. O. Berdel, D. Moore, et al., "Whole Body Vibration Therapy: A Novel Potential Treatment for Type 2 Diabetes Mellitus," *SpringerPlus* 4 (October 6, 2015):578, doi:10.1186/s40064-015-1373-0.

51. Mitch Leslie, "Good Vibrations: A Bit of Shaking Can Burn Fat, Combat Diabetes," *Science* (March 15, 2017), doi:10.1126/science.aal0919.

52. Barbara Bolen, "The Role Dysbiosis May Be Playing in Your Health", *Verywell Health* online (updated August 14, 2019), https://www.verywellhealth.com /what-is-intestinal-dysbiosis-1945045.

53. J. C. Yu, V. L. Hale, H. Khodadadi, and B. Baban, "Whole Body Vibration-Induced Omental Macrophage Polarization and Fecal Microbiome Modification in a Murine Model," *International Journal of Molecular Sciences* 20, no. 13 (June 26, 2019): e3125, doi:10.3390/ijms20133125.

Chapter 3

1. Patrick L. Barry, "Good Vibrations: A New Treatment under Study by NASA-Funded Doctors Could Reverse Bone Loss Experienced by Astronauts in Space," NASA, https://web.archive.org/web/20020209180125/http://science.nasa.gov /headlines/y2001/ast02nov_1.htm.

2. Ibid.

3. Gina Kolata, "Low Buzz May Give Mice Better Bones and Less Fat." *New York Times* 30 (October 30, 2007), https://www.nytimes.com/2007/10/30/health /research/30bone.html?_r=1.

4. A. Prioreschi, T. Oosthuyse, I. Avidon, and J. McVeigh, "Whole Body Vibration Increases Hip Bone Mineral Density in Road Cyclists." *International Journal of Sports Medicine* 33, no. 8 (August 2012): 593–9, doi:10.1055/s-0032-1301886.

5. P. Y. Liu, K. Brummel-Smith, and J. Z. Ilich, "Aerobic Exercise and Whole-Body Vibration in Offsetting Bone Loss in Older Adults," *Journal of Aging Research* (January 3, 2011):379674, doi:10.4061/2011/379674.

6. J. O. Totosy de Zepetnek, L. M. Giangregorio, and B. C. Craven, Whole-Body Vibration as Potential Intervention for People with Low Bone Mineral Density and Osteoporosis: A Review," *Journal of Rehabilitation Research and Development* 46, no. 4 (2009):529–42.

7. L. Slatkovska, S. M. Alibhai, J. Beyene, et al., "Effect of 12 Months of Whole-Body Vibration Therapy on Bone Density and Structure in Postmenopausal Women: A Randomized Trial," *Annals of Internal Medicine* 155, no. 10 (November 15, 2011):668–79, W205, doi:10.7326/0003-4819-155-10-201111150-00005.

8. C. Rubin, R. Recker, D. Cullen, et al., "Prevention of Postmenopausal Bone Loss by a Low-Magnitude, High-Frequency Mechanical Stimuli: A Clinical Trial Assessing Compliance, Efficacy, and Safety," *Journal of Bone and Mineral Research* 19, no. 3 (2004):343–51, doi:10.1359/JBMR.0301251.

9. C. L. Lai, S. Y. Tseng, C. N. Chen, et al., "Effect of 6 Months of Whole Body Vibration on Lumbar Spine Bone Density in Postmenopausal Women: A Randomized Controlled Trial," *Clinical Interventions in Aging* 8 (2013):1603–9 doi:10.2147/CIA.S53591.

10. Elena Marín-Cascales, P. E. Alcaraz, D. J. Ramos-Campo, et al., "Whole-Body Training and Bone Health in Postmenopausal Women: A Systematic Review and Meta-Analysis," *Medicine (Baltimore)* 97, no. 34 (August 2018): e11918, doi:10.1097/MD.0000000000011918.

11. Ibid.

12. Slatkovska et al., "Effect of 12 Months of Whole-Body Vibration."

13. Rubin et al., "Prevention of Postmenopausal Bone Loss."

14. Marín-Cascales et al., "Whole-Body Training and Bone Health in Postmenopausal Women." ı."

15. Ibid. n."

Chapter 4

1. "Meditation: A Pathway to Pain Relief," *Practical Pain Management* online (updated 2/07/17), https://www.practicalpainmanagement.com/patient/treatments /alternative/meditation-pathway-pain-relief. Original source: F. Zeidan, A. L. Adler-Neal, R. E, Wells, et al., "Mindfulness-Meditation-Based Pain Relief Is Not Mediated by Endogenous Opioids," *Journal of Neuroscience* 36, no. 11 (2016): 3391–3397.

2. Y. Zheng, X. Wang, B. Chen, et al., "Effect of 12-Week Whole-Body Vibration Exercise on Lumbopelvic Proprioception and Pain Control in Young Adults with Nonspecific Low Back Pain," *Medical Science Monitor* 25 (2019): 443–452, doi:10.12659/msm.912047.

3. B. del Pozo-Cruz, M. A. Hernández Mocholí, J. C. Adsuar, et al., "Effects of Whole Body Vibration Therapy on Main Outcome Measures for Chronic Non-Specific Low Back Pain: A Single-Blind Randomized Controlled Trial," *Journal of Rehabilitation Medicine* 43, no. 8 (July 2011): 689–94, doi:10.2340/16501977-0830.

4. T. S. Kaeding, A. Karch, R. Schwarz, et al., "Whole-Body Vibration Training as a Workplace-Based Sports Activity for Employees with Chronic Low-Back Pain," *Scandinavian Journal of Medicine and Science in Sports* 27, no. 12 (2017): 2027–39, doi:10.1111/sms.12852.

5. J. Rittweger, K. Just, K. Kautzsch, et al., "Treatment of Chronic Lower Back Pain with Lumbar Extension and Whole-Body Vibration Exercise: A Randomized Controlled Trial," *Spine* 27, no. 17 (September 2002): 1829–34, doi:10.1097/00007632-200209010-00003.

6. Ibid.

7. A. Elfering, J. Zahno, J. Taeymans, et al., "Acute Effects of Stochastic Resonance Whole Body Vibration," *World Journal of Orthopedics* 4, no. 4 (October 18, 2013): 291–8, doi:10.5312/wjo.v4.i4.291.

8. J. Bidonde, A. J. Busch, I. van der Spuy, et al., "Whole Body Vibration Exercise Training for Fibromyalgia," *Cochrane Database of Systematic Reviews* 9 (September 2017): CD011755, doi:10.1002/14651858.CD011755.pub2.

9. H. R. Bokaeian, A. H. Bakhtiary, M. Mirmohammadkhani, and J. Moghimi, "The Effect of Adding Whole Body Vibration Training to Strengthening Training in the Treatment of Knee Osteoarthritis: A Randomized Clinical Trial," *Journal of Bodywork and Movement Therapies* 20, no. 2 (April 2016): 334–340, doi:10.1016/j.jbmt.2015.08.005,.

10. Y. G. Park, B. S. Kwon, J. W. Park, et al., "Therapeutic Effect of Whole Body Vibration on Chronic Knee Osteoarthritis," *Annals of Rehabilitation Medicine* 37, no. 4 (August 2013):505–15, doi:10.5535/arm.2013.37.4.505.

11. A. P. Simão, N. C. Avelar, R. Tossige-Gomes, et al., "Functional Performance and Inflammatory Cytokines After Squat Exercises and Whole-Body Vibration in Elderly Individuals with Knee Osteoarthritis," *Archives of Physical Medicine and Rehabilitation* 93, no. 10 (2012): 1692–1700, doi:10.1016/j.apmr.2012.04.017.

12. Bokaeian et al., "The Effect . . . in the Treatment of Knee Osteoarthritis."

13. Park et al., "Therapeutic Effect . . . on Chronic Knee Osteoarthritis."

14. Simão et al., "Functional Performance and Inflammatory Cytokines."

15. T. Tsuji, J. Yoon, T. Aiba, A. Kanamori, et al., "Effects of Whole-Body Vibration Exercise on Muscular Strength and Power, Functional Mobility and Self-Reported Knee Function in Middle-Aged and Older Japanese Women with Knee Pain," *Knee* 21, no. 6 (December 2014): 1088–1095, doi:10.1016/j .knee.2014.07.015.

16. T. Trans, J. Aaboe, M. Henriksen, R. Christensen, et al., "Effect of Whole Body Vibration Exercise on Muscle Strength and Proprioception in Females with Knee Osteoarthritis," *Knee* 16, no. 4 (August 2009): 256–61, doi:10.1016/j .knee.2008.11.014.

17. N. C. Avelar, A. P. Simão, R. Tossige-Gomes, C. D. Neves, et al., "The Effect of Adding Whole-Body Vibration to Squat Training on the Functional Performance and Self-Report of Disease Status in Elderly Patients with Knee Osteoarthritis: A Randomized, Controlled Clinical Study," *Journal of Alternative*

and *Complementary Medicine* 17, no. 12 (2011): 1149–1155, doi:10.1089/acm.2010.0782.

18. H. Zafar, A. Alghadir, S. Anwer, and E. Al-Eisa, "Therapeutic Effects of Whole-Body Vibration Training in Knee Osteoarthritis: A Systematic Review and Meta-Analysis," *Archives of Physical Medicine and Rehabilitation* 96, no. 8 (2015): 1525–1532, doi:10.1016/j.apmr.2015.03.010.

19. Ibid.

20. P. Wang, X. Yang, Y. Yang, L. Yang, et al., "Effects of Whole Body Vibration on Pain, Stiffness and Physical Functions in Patients with Knee Osteoarthritis: A Systematic Review and Meta-Analysis," *Clinical Rehabilitation* 29, no. 10 (2015): 939–51, doi:10.1177/0269215514564895.

21. Simão et al., "Functional Performance and Inflammatory Cytokines."

22. V. G. C. Ribeiro, V. A. Mendonça, A. L. C. Souza, et al., "Inflammatory Biomarkers Responses After Acute Whole Body Vibration in Fibromyalgia," *Brazilian Journal of Medical and Biological Research* 51, no. 4 (March 2018): e6775, doi:10.1590/1414-431X20176775.

23. Meghan McGee-Lawrence, K. H. Wenger, S. Misra, et al., "Whole-Body Vibration Mimics the Metabolic Effects of Exercise in Male Leptin Receptor-Deficient Mice," *Endocrinology* 158, no. 5 (May 1, 2017): 1160–1171, doi:10.1210/en.2016-1250.

24. E. Alentorn-Geli, J. Padilla, G. Moras, et al., "Six Weeks of Whole-Body Vibration Exercise Improves Pain and Fatigue in Women with Fibromyalgia," *Journal of Alternative and Complementary Medicine* 14, no. 8 (October 2008): 975–81, doi:10.1089/acm.2008.0050.

25. Bokaeian et al., "The Effect . . . in the Treatment of Knee Osteoarthritis."

26. Zheng et al., "Effect of 12-Week Whole-Body Vibration Exercise on Lumbopelvic Proprioception."

27. N. Schneiderman, G. Ironson, and S. D. Siegel, "Stress and Health: Psychological, Behavioral, and Biological Determinants," *Annual Review of Clinical Psychology* 1 (2005): 607–628, doi:10.1146/annurev.clinpsy.1.102803.144141.

28. Marin-Cascales et al., "Effects of 24 Weeks of Whole Body Vibration."

Chapter 5

1. Gretchen Reynolds, "Jogging Your Brain," *New York Times* magazine (April 2012): 46.

2. Sang-Soo Kim, Sung-Bum Ju, and Gi Duck Park, "Changes in Stress Hormone Levels with the Application of Vibrations before Resistance Exercises at Different Intensities," *Journal of Physical Therapy Science* 27, no. 9 (2015): 2845–2847, doi:10.1589/jpts.27.2845.

3. M. Ariizumi and A. Okada, "Effect of Whole Body Vibration on the Rat Brain Content of Serotonin and Plasma Corticosterone," *European Journal of Applied Physiology and Occupational Physiology* 52, no. 1 (1983): 15–9, doi:10.1007/bf00429019.

4. S. Sharififar, R. A. Coronado, S. Romero, et al., "The Effects of Whole Body Vibration on Mobility and Balance in Parkinson Disease: A Systematic Review," *Iranian Journal of Medical Sciences* 39, no. 4 (July 2014): 318–326.

5. S. D. Santos-Filho, M. H. Cameron, and M. Bernardo-Filho, "Benefits of Whole-Body Vibration with an Oscillating Platform for People with Multiple Sclerosis: A Systematic Review," *Multiple Sclerosis International* (2012): 274728, doi:10.1155/2012/274728.

6. E. D. S. Freitas, C, Frederiksen, R. M. Miller, et al., "Acute and Chronic Effects of Whole-Body Vibration on Balance, Postural Stability, and Mobility in Women with Multiple Sclerosis," *Dose Response* 16, no. 4 (December 27, 2018): 1559325818816577, doi:10.1177/1559325818816577.

7. M. Fischer, T. Vialleron, G. Laffaye, et al., "Long-Term Effects of Whole-Body Vibration on Human Gait: A Systematic Review and Meta-Analysis," *Frontiers in Neurology* 10 (June 19, 2019): 627, doi:0.3389/fneur.2019.00627.

8. G. Ebersbach, D. Edler, O. Kaufhold, and J. Wissel, "Whole Body Vibration versus Conventional Physiotherapy to Improve Balance and Gait in Parkinson's Disease," *Archives of Physical Medicine and Rehabilitation* 89, no. 3 (March 2008): 399–403, doi:10.1016/j.apmr.2007.09.031.

9. Anne Trafton, "Synchronized Brain Waves Enable Rapid Learning: MIT Study Finds Neurons That Hum Together Encode New Information," MIT News Office online (June 12, 2014), http://news.mit.edu/2014/synchronized-brain-waves-enable-rapid-learning-0612.

10. Ibid.

11. Ibid.

12. J. Dispenza, *Becoming Supernatural: How Common People are Doing the Uncommon* (Carlsbad, CA: Hay House, 2017), 67.

13. Ibid., 65–67.

14. Ervin Lazlo, *You Can Change the World: The Global Citizen's Handbook for Living on Planet Earth* (New York: SelectBooks, 2003).

15. Norman Shealy, *Soul Medicine* (Santa Rosa, CA: Elite Books, 2006), 208–212.

16. L. Song, G. Schwartz, and L. Russek, "Heart-Focused Attention and Heart-Brain Synchronization: Energetic and Physiological Mechanisms," *Alternative Therapies in Health and Medicine* 4, no. 5 (1998): 44–52, 54–60, 62.

17. D. L. Childre, H. Martin, and D Beech, *The HeartMath Solution: The Institute of HeartMath's Revolutionary Program for Engaging the Power of the Heart's Intelligence* (San Francisco: HarperSanFrancisco, 1999), 33.

18. Dispenza, *Becoming Supernatural*, 33.

19. Richard Gerber, *Vibrational Medicine*, 3rd ed. (Rochester, NY: Bear and Co., 2001), 53–56.

20. Shealy, *Soul Medicine*, 212.

21. Ibid., 213.

22. Ibid., 212.

23. L. Terhorst, M. J. Schneider, K. H. Kim, et al., "Complementary and Alternative Medicine in the Treatment of Pain in Fibromyalgia: A Systematic Review of Randomized Controlled Trials," *Journal of Manipulative and Psychological Therapeutics* 34, no. 7 (September 2011: 483–96), doi:10.1016/j.jmpt.2011.05.006.

24. Richard Gerber, *Vibrational Medicine: The #1 Handbook of Subtle-Energy Therapies* (Rochester, VT: Bear & Co., 2001).

25. N. M. Dhanani, T. J. Caruso, and A. J. Carinci, "Complementary and Alternative Medicine for Pain: An Evidence-Based Review," *Current Pain and Headache Reports* 15, no.1 (February 2011): 39–46, doi:10.1007/s11916-010-0158-y.

26. J. M. Day and A. J. Nitz, "The Effect of Muscle Energy Techniques on Disability and Pain Scores in Individuals with Low Back Pain," *Journal of Sport Rehabilitation* 21, no. 2 (May 2012): 194–8.

27. Bill Reddy, "Insights with Norm Shealy," *Acupuncture Today* 13, no. 6 (June 2012), https://www.acupuncturetoday.com/mpacms/at/article.php?id=32580.

28. Keith DeOrio, *Vibranetics: The Complete Whole Body Vibration Fitness Solution* (Santa Monica, CA: self-published, 2008), 31.

Chapter 6

1. C. Bosco, M. Iacovelli, O. Tsarpela, et al., "Hormonal Responses to Whole-Body Vibration in Men," *European Journal of Applied Physiology* 81, no. 6 (April 2000): 449–454, doi:10.1007/s004210050067.

2. Lev G. Fedyniak, "Can Your Cat's Purr Heal?" *Animal Wellness* (September 2010), https://animalwellnessmagazine.com/cats-purr-heal.

3. Bosco et al., "Hormonal Responses."

4. M. Giunta, M. Cardinale, F. Agosti, et al., "Growth Hormone-Releasing Effects of Whole Body Vibration Alone or Combined with Squatting Plus External Load in Severely Obese Female Subjects," *Obesity Facts* 5, no. 4 (August 2012): 567–574, doi:10.1159/000342066.

5. A. Sartorio, F. Agosti, A. De Col, et al., "Growth Hormone and Lactate Responses Induced by Maximal Isometric Voluntary Contractions and Whole-Body Vibrations in Healthy Subjects," *Journal of Endocrinological Investigation* 34, no. 3, (March 2011): 216–221, doi:10.3275/7255.

6. S. Murphy, K. T. Khaw, A. Cassidy, and J. E. Compston, "Sex Hormones and Bone Mineral Density in Elderly Men," *Bone and Mineral* 20, no. 2 (1993): 133–40.

7. T. Kvorning, M. Bagger, P. Caserotti, and K. Madsen, "Effects of Vibration and Resistance Training on Neuromuscular and Hormonal Measures," *European Journal of Applied Physiology* 96, no. 5 (March 2006): 615–625, doi:10.1007/s00421-006-0139-3.

8. Susan Rako, *The Hormone of Desire: The Truth about Testosterone, Sexuality, and Menopause* (New York: Three Rivers Press, 1996), 25.

9. http://www.rxlist.com/androgel-side-effects-drug-center.htm.

10. Bosco et al., "Hormonal Responses."

11. Murphy et al., "Sex Hormones and Bone Mineral Density."

12. P. J. Kelly, N. A. Pocock, P. N. Sambrook, and J. A. Eisman, "Dietary Calcium, Sex Hormones, and Bone Mineral Density in Men," *British Medical Journal* 300, no. 6736 (May 26, 1990): 1361–4, doi:10.1136/bmj.300.6736.1361.

13. G. A. Greendale, S. Edelstein, and E. Barrett-Connor, "Endogenous Sex Steroids and Bone Mineral Density in Older Women and Men: The Rancho Bernardo Study," *Journal of Bone and Mineral Research* 12, no. 11 (1997): 1833–43, doi:10.1359/jbmr.1997.12.11.1833.

14. Giunta et al., "Growth Hormone-Releasing Effects."

15. Sartorio et al., "Growth Hormone and Lactate Responses."

16. Kvorning et al., "Effects of Vibration and Resistance Training."

17. Bosco et al., "Hormonal Responses."

18. Kvorning et al., "Effects of Vibration and Resistance Training."

19. Giunta et al., "Growth Hormone-Releasing Effects."

20. Sartorio et al., "Growth Hormone and Lactate Responses."

21. Fischer et al., "Long-Term Effects of Whole-Body Vibration on Human Gait."

22. Ibid.

23. Ibid.

Chapter 7

1. R. Tossige-Gomes, N. C. Avelar, A. P. Simão, et al., "Whole-Body Vibration Decreases the Proliferative Response of TCD4+ Cells in Elderly Individuals with Knee Osteoarthritis," *Brazilian Journal of Medical and Biological Research* 45, no. 12 (December 2012): 1262–1268, doi:10.1590/S0100-879X2012007500139.

2. J. C. Yu, V. L. Hale, H. Khodadadi, and B. Baban, "Whole Body Vibration-Induced Omental Macrophage Polarization and Fecal Microbiome Modification in a Murine Model," *International Journal of Molecular Sciences* 20, no. 13 (June 26, 2019): e3125, doi:10.3390/ijms20133125.

3. "Chemical Body Burden," test results done on Bill Moyers by Dr. Michael McCally, http://www.pbs.org/tradesecrets/problem/bodyburden.html.

4. Sherry A. Rogers, *Detoxify or Die* (Sarasota, FL: Sand Key Co., 2002), 89.

Chapter 9

1. Y. Zheng, X. Wang, B. Chen, et al., "Effect of 12-Week Whole-Body Vibration Exercise on Lumbopelvic Proprioception and Pain Control in Young Adults with Nonspecific Low Back Pain," *Medical Science Monitor* 25 (2019): 443–452, doi:10.12659/msm.912047.

2. B. del Pozo-Cruz, M. A. Hernández Mocholí, J. C. Adsuar, et al., "Effects of Whole Body Vibration Therapy on Main Outcome Measures for Chronic Non-Specific Low Back Pain: A Single-Blind Randomized Controlled Trial," *Journal of Rehabilitation Medicine* 43, no. 8 (July 2011): 689–94, doi:10.2340/16501977-0830.

3. T. S. Kaeding, A. Karch, R. Schwarz, et al., "Whole-Body Vibration Training as a Workplace-Based Sports Activity for Employees with Chronic Low-Back Pain," *Scandinavian Journal of Medicine and Science in Sports* 27, no. 12 (2017): 2027–39, doi:10.1111/sms.12852.

4. J. Rittweger, K. Just, K. Kautzsch, et al., "Treatment of Chronic Lower Back Pain with Lumbar Extension and Whole-Body Vibration Exercise: A Randomized Controlled Trial," *Spine* 27, no. 17 (September 2002): 1829–34, doi:10.1097/00007632-200209010-00003.

ADDITIONAL RESEARCH STUDIES

Bone Density

Beck, B. R., and T. L. Norling. "The Effect of 8 Months of Twice-Weekly Low- or Higher Intensity Whole Body Vibration on Risk Factors for Postmenopausal Hip Fracture." *American Journal of Physical Medicine and Rehabilitation* 89, no. 12 (2010): 997–1009. doi:10.1097/PHM.0b013e3181f71063.

Davis, Ronald, James Rowe, David L. Nichols, et al. "Effects of Two Intensities of Whole Body Vibration on Fall-Related Risk Factors in Postmenopausal Women." *Journal of Women's Health, Issues, and Care* 3, no. 6 (2014): 2. doi:10.4172/2325-9795.1000167.

Felman, Adam (reviewed by Justin Choi, MD). "Everything You Need to Know about Inflammation." Medical News Today online. Last updated November 24, 2017. www.medicalnewstoday.com/articles/248423.php.

Gómez-Cabello, A., I. Ara, A. González-Agüero, et al. "Effects of Training on Bone Mass in Older Adults: A Systematic Review." *Sports Medicine* 42, no. 4 (2012): 301–25. doi:10.2165/11597670-000000000-00000.

Grossman, P., L. Niemann, S. Schmidt, and H. Walach. "Mindfulness-Based Stress Reduction and Health Benefits: A Meta-Analysis." *Journal of Psychosomatic Research* 57, no. 1 (July 2004): 35–43. doi:10.1016/S0022-3999(03)00573-7.

Karakiriou, S. K., H. T. Douda, I. G. Smilios, and K. A. Volaklis. "Effects of Vibration and Exercise Training on Bone Mineral Density and Muscle Strength in Postmenopausal Women." *European Journal of Sport Science* 12, no. 1 (2012): 81–8. doi:10.1080/17461391.2010.536581.

Liphardt, A. M., J. Schipilow, D. A. Hanley, and S. K. Boyd. "Bone Quality in Osteopenic Postmenopausal Women Is Not Improved after 12 Months of Whole-Body Vibration Training." *Osteoporosis International* 26, no. 3 (2015): 911–20. doi:10.1007/s00198-014-2995-8.

Ruan, X. Y., F. Y. Jin, Y. L. Liu, et al. "Effects of Vibration Therapy on Bone Mineral Density in Postmenopausal Women with Osteoporosis." *Chinese Medical Journal* 21, no. 13 (July 5, 2008): 1155–8.

Verschueren, S. M., M. Roelants, C. Delecluse, et al. "Effect of 6-Month Whole Body Vibration Training on Hip Density, Muscle Strength, and Postural Control in Postmenopausal Women: A Randomized Controlled Pilot Study." *Journal of Bone and Mineral Research* 19, no. 3 (2004): 352–9. doi:10.1359/JBMR.0301245.

Von Stengel, S., W. Kemmler, M. Bebenek, et al. "Effects of Whole-Body Vibration Training on Different Devices on Bone Mineral Density." *Medicine and Science in Sports and Exercise* 43, no. 6 (2011): 1071–9. doi:10.1249/MSS.0b013e318202f3d3.

Wegner, M., I. Helmich, S. Machado, et al. "Effects of Exercise on Anxiety and Depression Disorders: Review of Meta-Analyses and Neurobiological Mechanisms." *CNS & Neurological Disorders Drug Targets* 13, no. 6 (2014): 1002–14.

Zeidan, F., A. L. Adler-Neal, R. E. Wells, et al. "Mindfulness-Meditation-Based Pain Relief Is Not Mediated by Endogenous Opioids." *Journal of Neuroscience* 36, no. 11 (March 16, 2016): 3391–3397. doi:10.1523/jneurosci.4328-15.2016.

Brain Synchronization

Abraha, I., F. Trotta, J. M. Rimland, A. Cruz-Jentoft, et al. "Efficacy of Non-Pharmacological Interventions to Prevent and Treat Delirium in Older Patients: A Systematic Overview. The SENATOR project ONTOP Series." *PLoS ONE* 10, no. 6 (2015): e1023090. doi:10.1371/journal.pone.0123090.

Danilenko, K. V., and I. A. Ivanova. "Dawn Simulation vs. Bright Light in Seasonal Affective Disorder: Treatment Effects and Subjective Preference." *Journal of Affective Disorders* 180 (July 15, 2015): 87–9. doi:10.1016/j.jad.2015.03.055.

da Silva, V. F., A. P. Ribeiro, V. A. Dos Santos, A. E. Nardi, A. L. King, and M. R. Calomeni. "Stimulation by Light and Sound: Therapeutics Effects in Humans: Systematic Review." *Clinical Practice and Epidemiology in Mental Health* 11 (June 26, 2015): 150–54. doi:10.2174/1745017901511010150.

Petrovsky, D., P. Z. Cacchione, and M. George. "Review of the Effect of Music Interventions on Symptoms of Anxiety and Depression in Older Adults with Mild Dementia." *International Psychogeriatrics* 27, no. 10 (April 29, 2015): 1–10. doi:10.1017/S1041610215000393.

Raglio, A., C. Galandra, L. Sibilla, F. Esposito, et al. "Effects of Active Music Therapy on the Normal Brain: fMRI Based Evidence." *Brain Imaging and Behavior* 10, no. 1 (March 2016): 182–6. doi:10.1007/s11682-015-9380-x.

Schwartz, R. S., and J. Olds. "The Psychiatry of Light." *Harvard Review of Psychiatry* 23, no. 3 (May/June 2015): 188–94. doi:10.1097/HRP.0000000000000078.

Shealy, C. N. "The Reality of EEG and Neurochemical Responses to Photostimulation: Part I." In *Light Years Ahead: The Illustrated Guide to Full Spectrum and Colored Light in Mindbody Healing,* edited by Brian Breiling. Berkeley: Celestial Arts Press, 1996.

———. "The Reality of EEG and Neurochemical Responses to Photostimulation: Part II." In *Light Years Ahead: The Illustrated Guide to Full Spectrum and Colored Light in Mindbody Healing,* edited by Brian Breiling. Berkeley: Celestial Arts Press, 1996.

———, R. K. Cady, D. C. Veehoff, M. Burnetti-Atwell, et al. "Effects of Color Photostimulation upon Neurochemicals and Neurohormones." *Journal of Neurological and Orthopaedic Medicine and Surgery* 17, no. 1 (1996): 95–96.

———, T. L. Smith, P. Thomlinson, and W. A. Tiller. "A Double-Blind EEG Response Test for a Supposed Electromagnetic Field-Neutralizing Device. Part I: Via the Clinician Expertise Procedure." *Subtle Energies and Energy Medicine* 9, no. 3, 231–45.

Sun J., and W. Chen. "Music Therapy for Coma Patients: Preliminary Results." *European Review for Medical and Pharmacological Sciences* 19, no. 7 (April 2015): 1209–18.

Candida Yeast

Chaitow, Leon. *Candida Albicans: Could Yeast Be Your Problem?* Rochester, VT: Healing Arts Press, 1998.

Crook, William. *The Yeast Connection: A Medical Breakthrough*. Berkeley, CA: Crown Publishing Group, 1994

Trowbridge, John Parks, and Morton Walker. *The Yeast Syndrome*. New York: Bantam Books, 1985.

Wunderlich, Ray Jr., and Dwight Kalita. *The Candida Yeast Syndrome*. New York: McGraw-Hill, 1998.

Meditation

Tlalka, Stephany. "Meditation Is the Fastest Growing Health Trend in America." *Health* (December 11, 2018). https://mindful.org.

Zeidan, F., and D. R. Vago. "Mindfulness Meditation-Based Pain Relief: A Mechanistic Account." *Annals of the New York Academy of Sciences* 1373, no. 1 (June 2016): 114–27. doi:10.1111/nyas.13153.

Neurological Diseases

del Pozo-Cruz, B., J. D. Adsuar, J. A. Parraca, et al. "Using Whole-Body Vibration Training in Patients Affected with Common Neurological Diseases: A Systematic Literature Review." *Journal of Alternative and Complementary Medicine* 18, no. 1 (2012): 29–41. doi:10.1089/acm.2010.0691.

Lee, G. "Whole-Body Vibration in Horizontal Direction for Stroke Rehabilitation: A Randomized Controlled Trial." *Medical Science Monitor* 25 (March 2019): 1621–1628. doi:10.12659/MSM.912589.

Ritzmann, R., C. Stark, and A. Krause. "Vibration Therapy in Patients with Cerebral Palsy: A Systematic Review." *Neuropsychiatric Disease and Treatment* 14 (June 18, 2018): 1607–1625. doi:10.2147/NDT.S152543.

Tupimai, T., P. Peungsuwan, J. Prasertnoo, J. Yamauchi. "Effect of Combining Passive Muscle Stretching and Whole Body Vibration on Spasticity and Physical Performance of Children and Adolescents with Cerebral Palsy." *Journal of Physical Therapy Science* 28, no.1 (Jan 30, 2016 Jan): 7–13. doi:10.1589/jpts.28.7.

About the Author

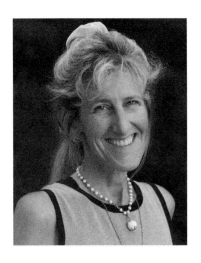

Becky Chambers is a natural health practitioner, teacher, author, and the president and owner of Vibrant Health, where she specializes in the breakthrough body, mind, and energy therapy of whole body vibration and the energy-medicine system of homeopathy. Ms. Chambers is a world expert in whole body vibration with twenty years of experience using and promoting it worldwide as an exercise and therapeutic system. Her best-selling book on the subject, *Whole Body Vibration: The Future of Good Health*, was released in 2013. Becky has a bachelor of science degree in biology from the University of Massachusetts, a master's in education from Lesley College, and she graduated from Clayton College of Natural Health in 2003 with a graduate degree in natural health, specializing in homeopathy.

She has spent the last thirty years discovering powerful new energy therapies that have led to a transformation of her life on every level. She has published two other books: *Homeopathy Plus*

Whole Body Vibration, and a memoir (not currently in print), *Beyond the Great Abyss: A True Story of Transformation through Natural Health Breakthroughs*.

Please visit her website at www.BCVibrantHealth.com.